Anti-diuretic Hormone

Anti-diuretic Hormone

Mary L. Forsling

Eden Press

Published by

Eden Press
1538 Sherbrooke St. W., Ste. 201
Montreal, Quebec, Canada H3G 1L5

and

Lunesdale House
Hornby
Lancaster LA2 8NB, England

ISBN 0 904406 51 2

Printed in Great Britain by
A. Wheaton & Co., Exeter

FOREWORD

This book primarily concentrates on a detailed and critical discussion of work published in 1974 and 1975. Inevitably of course I have had to set the new findings in the context of the old and many earlier references are included. I hope that the result is a comprehensive and helpful account of the present state of knowledge. I apologise for any errors or omissions. I should be grateful to anyone who draws my attention to these.

I wish to thank friends both in the United Kingdom and the United States for valuable discussions. I also owe a debt of gratitude to my colleagues at the Middlesex Hospital Medical School, especially Felicity Boland, who played a great part in preparing the manuscripts.

Mary L. Forsling
Dept. of Physiology
Middlesex Hospital Medical School
London W1 7PN
England

August 1976

ANNUAL RESEARCH REVIEWS

Eden Press Annual Research Reviews are a new concept in medical and scientific publishing which will prove invaluable to research workers and to those interested in finding the latest information on a topic. Each review describes in detail the work published in one year on a particular topic, sets the new work in the context of the old and provides a near complete bibliography. Each topic is covered each year so that the successive annual volumes on any subject will provide a unique record of research in a field. The first volume in each series, while concentrating on the past year's work attempts to provide a "state of the art" account and also gives a bibliography of key earlier references. Each volume will be published within 3-4 months of receipt of the typescript.

Anyone interested in writing such an annual review in their own field should get in contact with the Series Editor, David F. Horrobin, Clinical Research Institute, 110 Pine Avenue West, Montreal, Quebec, Canada H2W lR7. Any topics either in medicine or in the basic medical sciences will be seriously considered. Titles already commissioned include Renin, Prolactin, Prostaglandins and the Kidney, Prostaglandins and the Gut, Regulation of Growth Hormone Secretion, Anti-diuretic Hormone, Somatostatin, Biofeedback, The Pineal, Duodenal Ulcer, Alcoholism, Rheumatoid Arthritis, Actions and Metabolism of Thyroid Hormones, Hodgkin's Disease and the Lymphomas, Schedule-induced Behaviour, Haemophilia, The Macrophage and Behaviour Therapy.

CONTENTS

Chapter 1

INTRODUCTION

"Just the place for a Snark! I have said it thrice:
What I tell you three times is true"

Interest in the neurohypophysis, as with most topics, is subject to cyclic variations. A few years ago attention to the neurohypophysis seemed to be on the wane, but recently there has been a resurgence of interest. Witness to this fact is the number of publications which have appeared on the subject. This review is based on the papers listed in *Index Medicus, Biological Abstract,* and *Chemical Abstracts,* from January to December 1975 and, during this time, the respective numbers of papers listed for vasopressin in each of these publications were 268, 362 and 233. There was less overlap between these abstracting services than one might imagine.

One factor contributing to this apparent revival of interest could be a possible parallelism between the cells of the neuroendocrine hypothalamus, producing releasing hormones and those of the paraventricular and supraoptic nuclei. Certainly a number of studies which have appeared on the pathways involved the mechanism of stimulus-secretion coupling. An interesting fact to emerge is that neurophysin-containing fibres pass not only to the posterior pituitary but also into the region of the median eminence, which raises again the question of whether vasopressin or neurophysin act as releasing factors. Another field of investigation has been the secretion of neurohypophysial hormones in the foetus.

At present, the mechanism of hormone action is exciting much attention and considerable effort has been devoted to elucidating the way in which vasopressin brings about changes in water permeability across amphibian membranes and in mammalian kidneys. Cyclic AMP has been shown to have a role and now evidence has appeared suggesting that microtubules may be involved.

One factor which has limited studies on the mechanisms of release of vasopressin was difficulty of assaying the hormone. A number of groups have now succeeded in establishing radioimmunoassays for vasopressin. However, very few of these assays have been extensively applied and it will be of interest to see whether this technique will contribute to our knowledge of the neurohypophysial system.

Synthesis of vasopressin and its analogues has now reached a fine art and attempts have been made to synthesise analogues possessing predominately either vasopressor or antidiuretic activity. Such analogues have proved to be of value in clinical practice. Inhibitors of vasopressin action could be of use in certain conditions and although such inhibitors have been synthesised, they have not been used clinically.

The term vasopressin is generally used in this review to denote arginine vasopressin, the antidiuretic hormone found in most mammalian species. The neurohypophysis was originally defined as that area including the neural lobe, median eminence and pituitary stalk. Recently, however, the term has been taken as being synonomous with the neural lobe or pars nervosa and this use will be adopted in the following chapters. Since it is a common experience in science that our Snarks turn out to be Boojums, each chapter is introduced by a quotation from *The Hunting of the Snark* (Carroll, 1876).

Chapter 2

LOCALISATION OF VASOPRESSIN AND NEUROPHYSIN SECRETING PATHWAYS

"And the crew were much pleased when
they found it to be
A map they could all understand."

Very extensive studies have been performed on the anatomy of the hypothalamo-hypophysial system and these have been reviewed by Knigge and Silverman (1974) who discussed the anatomy of the endocrine hypothalamus and Lederis (1974) who considered the structure of the system in terms of its neurosecretory function. That this complex represents a neurosecretory system was first demonstrated by Bargmann (1949) and Scharrer (1954). It clearly fulfills the criteria for a neurosecretory system - namely a system of neurones which produce a hormone or hormones and may thus be classified also as an endocrine system. The neurohypophysial system is amenable to study and has been used as a model for such systems. The investigations provide information on the endocrine hypothalamus which includes the magnocellular system itself. This latter comprises the supraoptic and paraventricular nuclei where oxytocin and vasopressin are synthesised together with so-called carrier proteins - the neurophysins. The hormones are packaged within neurosecretory granules, and are transported to the neural lobe where they are stored prior to release. In addition to supplying the neural lobe it has been suggested that the neurones from the supraoptic nucleus may also terminate in the median eminence.

It is generally considered that the supraoptic nucleus is largely concerned with the synthesis of vasopressin and the paraventricular nucleus with oxytocin. The neurosecretory nerve terminals contain two types of granules - dense core hormone containing granules 100-200 μ in diameter and smaller granules 50-60 μ in diameter, some of which may arise through rupture of membranes following secretion. There are also non-secretory nerve terminals in the posterior pituitary containing only small vesicles. Pituicytes, a type of glial cell, are also found in the posterior pituitary. Their function has not been proven, but they are thought to be involved in the secretory process.

Methods of Study of Hormone Secreting Pathways

In the work in which Bargmann first demonstrated the secretory nature of material produced by the magnocellular cells of the hypothalamus Gomori's chromealum - haematoxylin was used. Since then a number of different staining techniques have been employed including paraldehyde fuchsin which produces luminescence of neurosecretory material when observed under dark field conditions. More recently use has been made of immuno-fluorescence and immunochemistry. It is difficult to raise antisera to neurohypophysial hormones, but advantage has been taken of the antineurophysin antibodies which have been raised against recently purified neurophysins. It has been shown that there are several neurophysins including one which appears to be associated with vasopressin and one which seems specific for oxytocin. These specific peptides can be used as markers of hormone pathways.

Antibody complexed to a fluochrome may be used to locate cells containing a specific hormone. The covalent binding of the fluochrome to the antibody can frequently be an inefficient process, so to overcome this and other difficulties, the double antibody or sandwich technique is used. This technique, which has been used in the studies of Livert (1975) and Watkins (1975), entails initial treatment of the sections with rabbit antiserum raised against the peptide being studied (in this case neurophysin). Anti - rabbit - γ globulin antiserum labelled with fluorescein is then added, to visualise the position of the peptide, so that the rabbit γ globulin is effectively sandwiched between the neurophysin and the anti-rabbit globulin whilst the whole complex bears a fluorescent label.

Although a valuable technique, immunofluorescence has a number of disadvantages. Unfixed tissue is generally used so that the result is not permanent. Natural fluorescence of the tissue may interfere and the scattered light, arising from the section, renders fine resolution difficult. For these and other reasons immunochemical staining has been adopted (Watkins 1975; Zimmerman, Defendini, Sokol and Robinson, 1975). Both these groups of workers have used the three layer immunoperoxidase bridge technique. In this procedure hydrated sections are reacted successively with anti-neurophysin or anti-hormone serum (primary antiserum), rabbit γ globulin serum, rabbit antiperoxidase serum, peroxidase and finally 3'3 diaminobenzidine to demonstrate the peroxidase activity. Apart from preserving the tissue well, this method appears to be more sensitive than that of immunofluorescence. The primary antiserum to vasopressin which was used by Silverman and Zimmerman was raised in rabbits against lysine vasopressin coupled to bovine serum albumin. Such studies of the neurophysin pathways have been performed on the guinea pig (Silverman and Zimmerman, 1975), the mouse, the rat and the monkey (Zimmerman et al,

1975), the pig, the dog, the sheep (Watkins, 1975; Livett, 1975). Purified neurophysins from all these species have not been prepared, but there appear to be common antigenic determinants in many neurophysins so that a heterologous system may be used. Antisera to bovine, porcine, canine or human neurophysins have been used by the various authors listed.

Amongst other techniques available for identification of cells involved in the production of a given hormone is that of tissue culture of secretory cells with subsequent analysis of the hormonal product. In this context De Vitry, Camier Czernichow, Benda, Cohen and Tixier-Vidal (1974, 1975) have established a clone of mouse hypothalamic neurosecretory cells synthesizing neurophysin and vasopressin. The main use of this preparation of course is to study the regulation of the synthesis of neurohypophysin peptides (see Chapter 5).

Localisation of Neurophysin in the Mammalian Brain

Studies using the techniques described have most elegantly confirmed and extended the observations obtained with histochemical techniques. Immunoreactive neurophysin is found in considerable quantities in the large cells of the paraventricular and supraoptic nuclei indicating that this must be at the site of synthesis of the peptide. The neurophysin staining can be followed along the neuronal processes into the long axon and branching dendrites. Zimmerman et al (1975) report that the neurophysin-like material appears to be quite rapidly transferred along the axon, at a rate of 2.5 mm/h. Livett (1975) using immunofluorescence techniques was able to repeat earlier observations that neurosecretory material rapidly accumulates above the point where the hypothalamus-hypophysial tract is cut or abolished. Neurophysin is generally regarded as being solely present in the granules, but Silverman, Knigge and Zimmerman (1975), who describe a freeze-substitution technique for the neural lobe, saw an extragranular pool. This observation could be of importance in considering the release mechanisms of the hormones. It must however be treated with some caution as the technique precludes staining of intracellular membranes.

Another interesting observation to come from these histochemical methods, which are considerably more sensitive and specific than the Gomeri stains, is that the magnocellular system extends through a greater area in the hypothalamus than previously believed. Zimmerman et al found neurophysin in the infundibular nucleus. The differentiation of the magnocellular system into two distinct nuclei is not complete. This is especially true of the ox (Zimmerman et al 1975). The function of these two nuclei may therefore overlap. The question of the distribution of function of the two nuclei has been a subject of considerable debate.

Evidence for Separate Neurones

Bisset and his coworkers have shown that oxytocin and vasopressin can be separately released. It is not unreasonable therefore to suggest that the hormones themselves are produced in different neurones. Since the observation of Olivecrona (1975) that bilateral destruction of the paraventricular nuclei resulted in a loss of oxytocic activity in the posterior pituitary, much evidence has accumulated to suggest that the paraventricular nucleus is primarily concerned with production of oxytocin. Recent support for this hypothesis has come from Stutinsky (1974) studying transmitters in the hypothalamus. Further support has been provided by studies on the Brattleboro rat, an animal with an inherited inability to synthesise biologically active vasopressin. In order to throw more light on this question Zimmerman, Robinson, Husain and Acosta (1974) extracted tissue from the two nuclei on both sides of bovine hypothalamus and estimated the content of neurophysin I, neurophysin II, oxytocin and vasopressin. They demonstrated a clear relationship of neurophysin I to oxytocin and neurophysin II to vasopressin. It was suggested therefore that a specific neurophysin may be synthesized with each hormone. They also found that the ratio of vasopressin and oxytocin in the paraventricular nucleus was unity, but two to three in the supraoptic nucleus. Histological studies also revealed that the hormones were distributed between the two nuclei. Watkins (1975) showed that in DI rats there was hypertrophy of the magnocellular nuclei and that neurophysin was present in both the supraoptic and paraventricular nuclei in heterozygous and homozygous animals. Surprisingly he found evidence of material which cross-reacted with vasopressin antiserum. It is possible that the nuclei produced material with the amino acid sequence of the antigenic determinant, but no biological activity. Zimmerman et al made similar observations, demonstrating neurophysin in most cells of the supraoptic and paraventricular nuclei in control animals, whereas in the Battleboro rat only half the neurones in each of the nuclei contained neurophysin. They were further able to show that in the hypothalamus, oestrogen stimulated neurophysin (ESNP) and nicotine stimulated neurophysin (NSNP) were found in both supraoptic and paraventricular nuclei, but in different cell populations. Vandesande (1975), on the other hand, also using immunohistochemical techniques, has provided evidence that the supraoptic nucleus contains vasopressin, but felt that it was unlikely that these neurones also produced oxytocin. Livett was able to show in the pig that neurophysin II, the peptide preferentially associated with vasopressin was largely located in the supraoptic nucleus. Few positive staining cells were found in the paraventricular nucleus.

Burford, Dyball, Moss and Pickering (1974) have brought another technique to bear on the problem. They have injected ^{35}S - cysteine into one of the nuclei, or intracranially in rats with lesions in the other nucleus, and have followed incorporation into the two major neurophysins, one associated with vasopressin and one with oxytocin. When the label was injected into the paraventricular nucleus a relatively greater proportion of labelled oxytocin neurophysin was formed. Destruction of the paraventricular nucleus decreased the incorporation of label into this neurophysin. On the other hand ablation of the supraoptic nucleus resulted in less label being incorporated into the vasopressin neurophysin. Injection of ^{35}S - cysteine into the supraoptic nucleus gave equivocal results. The authors feel that this was because of the difficulties associated with injection into a flattened sheet of cells.

It would seem therefore that there are certain species differences but that the majority of vasopressin producing cells occur in the supraoptic nucleus although some are found in the paraventricular nucleus. Oxytocin-producing cells seem well distributed between the two nuclei. The question as to whether vasopressin and oxytocin are localised in the same or different neurones in the nuclei, remains unresolved.

Vasopressin and Neurophysin in the Median Eminence

Recently it has been shown in several species, (Silverman, Kozlowski, Zimmerman 1975; Zimmerman, Kozlowski, Scott, 1974; Livett, 1975; Watkins, 1975; Burlet, Marchetti, Duheille, 1974) that, in addition to the neurophysin staining material in the tracts leading from the hypothalamic nuclei to the posterior pituitary, some has been found in the external layer of the median eminence. Fibres appear to leave or branch from the main tract and pass to the external zone, ending around the portal capillaries. Vasopressin was also stained in these tracts in the rat and the mouse. This raises again the question of the possible use of neurohypophysial peptides in the release of the anterior pituitary hormones, especially ACTH. Indeed Watkins has suggested that the neurophysin-like material in the zona externa be named CRF associated neurophysin, since in adrenalectomy, when it is known that there is an increase in CRF, there is an increase in this neurophysin. The possibility that neurophysin is involved in the secretion of adenohypophysial hormone is, of course, highly speculative. It has been more frequently suggested that vasopressin is involved in the release of ACTH, either by potentiating the effect of CRF or by modulation of the portal system blood flow and membrane permeability. Neurophysin and vasopressin have been found in high concentrations in the portal blood of monkey, (Zimmerman, Carmel, Husain, Ferin, Tannenbaum, Frantz and Robinson, 1973).

Zimmerman et al (1975) have suggested that a second pathway is involved in the transport of neurohypophysial hormones to the portal blood. Neurophysin was demonstrated in the tanycytes in the area around the third ventricle, (Zimmerman, Kozlowski and Scott, 1974). Robinson and Zimmerman (1973) had previously shown that neurophysin was present in the CSF. These authors suggested that neurophysin, secreted from the fibres of the supra-optico-hypophysial systems into the CSF, was reabsorbed by the tanycytes and transported by their processes to the portal vessels (see Fig. 1). A similar mechanism has been proposed for the hypophysial releasing factors (Porter, Ben-Jonathan, Oliver, and Eskay, 1975). The recent studies of the neurosecretory system therefore have confirmed the observations made over the past 30 years. They have however re-opened the possible role of vasopressin in controlling ACTH release.

Summary and Conclusions

The nature of the hormone-secreting pathways has been determined using immunofluorescent and immunochemical techniques. Most investigations have been devoted to identifying the neurophysin-containing fibres. The studies have tended to confirm that each neurosecretory cell produces only one of the two neurohypophysial hormones. An interesting finding, which may cast vasopressin and neurophysin in a new role, is that some tracts pass to the region of the median eminence so that these peptides could pass into the portal capillaries supplying the anterior pituitary.

Figure 2.1

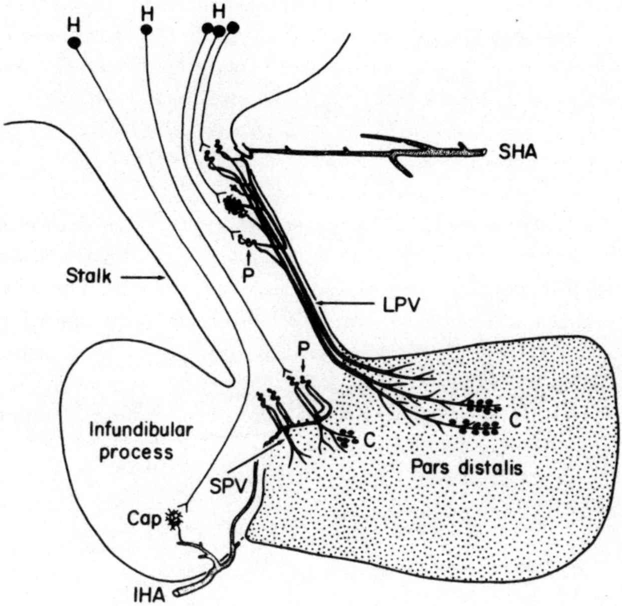

Diagram of the human pituitary in the sagittal plane.

H, or hypothalamic nuclei; I H A, S H A, inferior and superior hypophysial arteries; LPV, SPV, long and short portal vessels; P, primary capillary bed; cap, capillary bed; C, epithelial cells. [From P.M. Daniel and M.L. Prichard. Acta Endocrinol 80, Suppl 201, p 67, 1975. Reproduced with kind permission of the authors and publishers.]

Chapter 3

CHEMISTRY AND STRUCTURE-ACTIVITY RELATIONSHIPS

"Still keeping one principle object in view -
To preserve its symmetrical shape."

The mammalian antidiuretic hormone, arginine vasopressin (AVP) was isolated and the amino acid sequence determined by two independent groups (Du Vigneaud, Lawler and Popenoe, 1953; Acher and Chauvet, 1953). The amino acid sequence of vasopressin and oxytocin is shown in Fig. 3.1. It is only relatively recent however that attempts have been made to determine the tertiary structure (see e.g. Urry and Walter 1971; Walter, Smith and Deslaurirs 1974). The disulphide bridge between the amino acid residues at positions 11 and 6 is obviously a major determinant of the configuration of the molecule. Walter and his colleagues have proposed that the 20-membered ring of oxytocin forms a right-handed helical screw, the amino acids at positions 3 and 4 occupying the corners of the turn. They also propose a second turn in the linear portion of the molecule with the residues at 7 and 8 lying at the corners. The side chains of residues 3,4,7 and 8 therefore contribute little to the stability of the conformation of the molecule (Fig. 3.2).

Knowledge of the three-dimensional structure of a hormone is of course important in understanding its interaction with the receptor site. Structure-activity relationships have been studied using the 300 or so synthetic analogues which have been prepared. These studies followed the demonstration by Du Vigneaud and his coworkers in 1953 that the synthesis of physiologically active peptides is feasible. Preparation of these structural analogues represents an intriguing story in that some naturally occurring analogues were synthesized before they were discovered in nature. The amino acid substitutions in these naturally occurring analogues are at positions 3,4 and 8 which, as will be seen, have a relatively small effect on the stability of the peptide. Information derived from examination of the pituitary contents of many vertebrate species has provided a basis for speculation concerning the phylogenetic distribution of neurohypophysial hormones and the changes which they may have undergone during the course of evolution. It has been suggested (Acher, 1974) that the two naturally occurring molecules in the mammal have evolved from a common ancestral molecule, along two different lines, one being vasotocin - vasopressin and the other isotocin - mesotocin - oxytocin.

OXYTOCIN.

Cys - Tyr - Ileu[3] - Glu (NH_2) - Asp (NH_2) - Cys - Pro - Leu[8] - Gly (NH_2)
S ——— S (disulfide bridge Cys–Cys)

ARGININE-VASOPRESSIN.

Cys - Tyr - Phe[3] - Glu (NH_2) - Asp (NH_2) - Cys - Pro - Arg[8] - Gly (NH_2)
S ——— S

LYSINE-VASOPRESSIN.

Cys - Tyr - Phe[3] - Glu (NH_2) - Asp (NH_2) - Cys - Pro - Lys[8] - Gly (NH_2)
S ——— S

Figure 3.1. Sequence of amino acid residues in oxytocin and in arginine and lysine vasopressin.

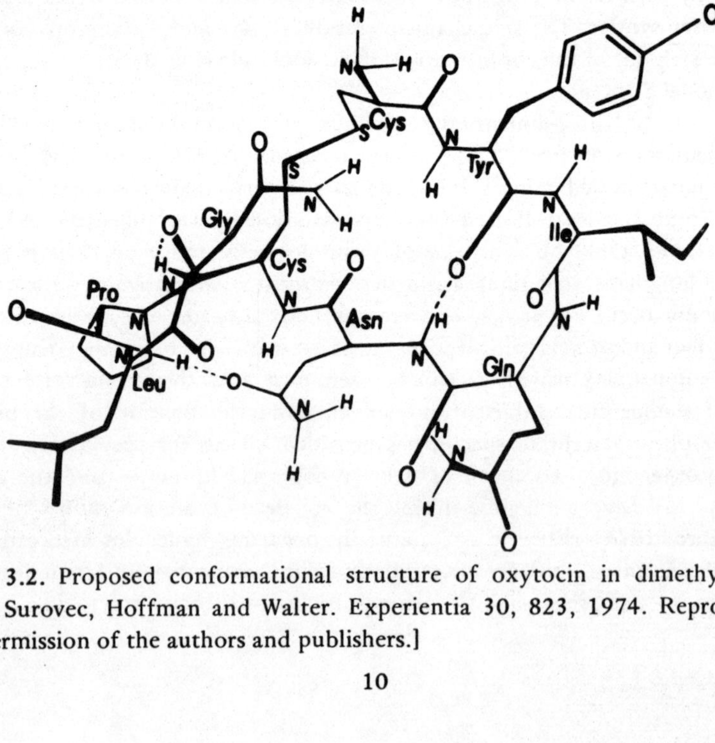

Figure 3.2. Proposed conformational structure of oxytocin in dimethylsulfoxide [From Surovec, Hoffman and Walter. Experientia 30, 823, 1974. Reproduced by kind permission of the authors and publishers.]

More recently the synthetic chemists have given their time to the synthesis of molecules for clinical use with a given spectrum of activity, e.g. low pressor and high antidiuretic activity or prolonged activity. The state of the art has reached a point where peptide synthesis is well-nigh routine and the problem of drug design can seriously be considered. This point is well illustrated in the theoretical approach adopted by Walter, Yamanaka and Sakakibara (1974) in the synthesis of a molecule with selective oxytocic activity and resistant to enzymic inactivation.

Synthesis of Vasopressin and Analogues

Solid phase synthesis of peptides, as described by Merrifield (1963), has been widely applied. The Peptide Hormone Group of the Shanghai Institute of Biochemistry (1975) have described a modification of this technique. The usual starting material for solid phase synthesis of peptides is chloromethylated polystyrene divinyl benzene which is reacted with an amino acid, in which the amino group is protected by a tert-butyloxycarbonyl (Boc) group, and triethylamine. The N-protected amino acid is thus bound to resin . The tert-butyloxycarbonyl group can then be removed and the product coupled with another Boc-amino acid. The above group of workers used the potassium salt of the N-protected amino acid instead of the triethyl ammonium salt. They claim that this improves the efficiency of esterification and so minimizes the formation of a quaternary anion exchanger which might cause side reactions as the synthesis progresses.

Conformational Structure

Walter, Ballardin, Schwartz, Gibbons and Wyssbrod, (1974) have now described studies in the conformation of arginine vasopressin and arginine vasotocin using the technique of proton magnetic resonance spectroscopy. They have shown that although there are certain significant differences in configuration from oxytocin, the overall back-bone arrangement is similar in dimethylsulphoxide . The conformational factor common to all naturally occurring mammalian principles is a ten-membered, hydrogen-bonded turn with the NH group of aspartic acid in position 5 bonded to the C=O grouping of tyrosine in position 2. There are however differences in the ring structure depending on the substitution. The C-terminal acrylic tail moiety possesses greater motility than the ring and in addition the tail of AVP shows greater motion than that of oxytocin.

In contrast to these studies using proton magnetic resonance spectroscopy, Fric, Kodicek, Flegel, Zaoral (1975) using circular dichroism studies found that freedom of the linear portion of oxytocin and vasopressin is similar. They suggest that the C-terminal is situated over the cyclic part of the molecule, thus allowing the tripeptide to interact with the primary aminogroup of cysteine. They also describe a face to face stacking of the tyrosine and phenylalanine side chains (in positions 2 and 3). This would put constraints on the conformational freedom of the tyrosine residue and probably distorts the dihedral angles of residues 1-3 of vasopressin as compared to oxytocin.

Klassen, Purdie, Lynn and Dioro (1974) have investigated the reaction of oxytocin and lysine vasopressin by pulse radiolysis. They found that reactivity effectively resides in the tyrosine, phenyl alanine and cysteine residues. The cyclic radical produced in the reaction is, as would be expected, more stable than the open chain sequence.

The studies of Smith, Clark, Ferger and Chan, (1975) on the synthetic analogue 3-β-(2-Thienyl)-alanine lysine vasopressin indicate that it is important for antidiuretic activity to have a hydrophobic aromatic side chain to residue 3. This peptide which they synthesised had enhanced antidiuretic potency with respect to lysine vasopressin, whereas the pressor potency was the same or slightly lower.

Analogues

Since the amino acids at positions 5,6 and 8 contribute little to the conformation of the molecules, Walter and his co-workers (Roy, Havran, Schwartz and Walter, 1975), have hypothesized that the amino acids at the corners of the turns participate in the hormone receptor interactions. Substitution in these positions should therefore affect the basal activity of these hormones. They have, indeed, shown this to be the case with oxytocin modified in positions 3 and 4. L-proline or D-alanine were substituted for the L-leucine residue in position 3 and in another series D-alanine or D-leucine were substituted for L-glutamine in position 4. All of these analogues showed profound reductions in biological activity.

Most current work on synthetic analogues is performed with the aim of modifying the biological spectrum of response by substitution as described above or of prolonging the activity by protecting the sites of enzymic attack. Vasopressin has two main types of activity - vasopressor and antidiuretic. Many analogues have been synthesised largely with a view to their clinical use, in which either one or the other activity has been enhanced. An analogue with enhanced antidiuretic activity which has been successfully used therapeutically is desamino-D-arginine vasopressin (DDAVP). In this analogue the terminal amino group has been removed and D-arginine substituted in the L-isomeric position 8, both of which manoevres improve antidiuretic potency. Estimates of the ratio of antidiuretic to pressor activity (A/P) vary, but a recent report gives a value of 238. The peptide however has only weak hydro-osmotic activity on the frog urinary bladder (Barth, LeBars, Roy and Jard, 1975). An analogue possessing enhanced pressor activity is ornithine vasopressin (POR – 8) in which the arginine residue is replaced by ornithine. This analogue is reported to have an A/P activity of 0.24.

During the course of 1975 several reports have appeared in which the clinical use of these two analogues has been described. Irmscher, Sennejunker, Wiegelman and Solbach (1974) studied the effects of DDAVP in 14 patients suffering from hypo thalamic diabetes insipidus. They found that, on a weight basis DDAVP produced a significantly more concentrated urine than LVP and that the duration of activity was ten times as long. Twenty four patients were given DDAVP intranasally for periods of up to 26 months and no side effects were observed. Nevertheless there was a reduced response to the drug at the end of this time. Nemethova and Lichardus (1974) have used the analogue in children and confirm its value therapeutically. Toursel and Fontaine (1975) have also used DDAVP in the treatment of pitressin-sensitive diabetes insipidus and Parkin (1975) found it of value for patients whose condition could not be controlled with lysine vasopressin. Apart from the potency of the compound, DDAVP is on the whole easier to administer than other forms of therapy, most of which have some drawbacks. Injections of pitressin tannate are painful and unpleasant in the long term. Nasal applications of pituitary preparations have been reported to give rise to allergic reactions. Lysine vasopressin nasal spray can result in nausea and dizziness and chlorpropamide is not suitable for use in children because of the risk of hypoglycaemia.

As DDAVP is easily administered, it was used by Aronson and Svenningsen (1974) to test the renal concentrating capacity in infants and children. This test obviates the somewhat hazardous procedure of dehydration. In most of the children DDAVP was administered intranasally. The maximum urinary concentrating ability using this drug was compared with that obtained with other widely used tests - the dehydration tests and pitressin. There was no significant difference in the maximum osmolality obtained in these various tests. The authors recommended the use of the DDAVP test which appears easy to perform and reliable. These same authors (Svenningsen and Aronson, 1974) have used the DDAVP test to follow the development of the renal concentrating capacity in normal healthy term and pre-term neonates and asphyxiated neonates. The tests were performed at 1 to 3 weeks of age and 4 to 6 weeks. Their results suggest that the renal concentrating capacity is not only influenced by maturity and anatomical growth, but possibly by extra-uterine need. A significantly lowered concentrating capacity was found in asphyxiated neonates in the first week or so of life. Thus, following perinatal asphyxia, tubular recovery appears to be delayed in relation to G.F.R.

There are obviously several clinical situations in which an analogue with basically pressor properties would be of value. Such haemostatic action would be of value in preventing bleeding from peptic ulcers, oesophageal varices (See Chapter 18) and the uterus and during various types of surgery such as the establishment of portocaval shunts in advanced cirrhosis. However most of the reports appearing during the year have concerned the use of POR 8 in maintaining haemostasis and a high concentration of local anaesthesia in facial and oral surgery. Mitrovic and Ristic (1974) used it successfully in 55 patients on whom various treatments were performed. They found no systemic cardiovascular effects following administration of the hormones and no post-operative haemorrhage or haematuria. Lindorf (1975) studied the effect of POR 8 using infra-red thermography. He found that the onset of vasoconstriction was slower than seen with adrenalin, but the duration of the effect was similar. In view of these results, Lindorf suggested that, as adrenalin may induce local acidosis and the combination of adrenalin with halogen-containing anaesthetics may bring about adverse cardiac reactions, the use of POR 8 may be preferable.

Waterson, (1975) too, feels that POR 8 may be of value in improving the effectiveness of local anaesthetic solutions. He used the perfused rabbit ear and the perfused rabbit ear artery to determine the potentiation by POR 8 of vascular responses to adrenalin. He found the constrictor responses to adrenalin in the rabbit ear were potentiated more than four fold by POR 8. He therefore suggested that the use of POR 8 could reduce the side effects of adrenalin by producing adequate vasoconstriction with lower doses of catecholamines given with the anaesthetic agent.

Structure - activity relationships of synthetic peptides

Apart from studies on those compounds already introduced into clinical practice, a number of investigations have been carried out on other synthetic analogues. Manning, Balaspiri, Judd, Acosta and Sawyer (1974) comment on substitutions affecting the antidiuretic specificity and duration of action. In addition to looking at the effect of deamination of position 1 and substitution of D-arginine for L-arginine as seen in DDAVP, they investigated the substitution of a more lipophilic residue in position 4. They report that the D-arginine substitution is the most important structural alteration as far as antidiuretic specificity is concerned. Substitution in position 4 is somewhat less effective, but still produces a decrease in the A/P ratio, sometimes by decreasing the vasopressor activity as is the case with valine, and aminobutyric acid. Deamination at position 1 had the least effect on antidiuretic specificity, but the greatest effect on the duration of activity. It has been speculated that this effect derives from the resistance of the peptides to metabolic degradation. Substitution of glutamine in position 4 by a more hydrophobic amino acid also had a pronounced effect on the length of action, the peptide having the longest action being 1-deamino-threonine.

A similar series of substitutions was looked at by Cort, Skopkova, Schuck, Stribrna and Sawyer (1973) and Jost, Procazka, Cort, Barth, Skopkova, Prusik and Sorm

(1974) who additionally substituted one sulphur in the disulphide bridge by CH_2, giving the carba derivatives. They carried out a non-D steric alteration of the C-terminal to give desamino-N-methyl arginine vasopressin. The carba derivatives were powerful antidiuretics but the steric dislocation of the back-bone produced by alteration at position 8, as in this last mentioned derivative, reduced the antidiuretic activity to one tenth that of AVP. These workers also considered the effect of the analogues on blood vessels. It appears that introducing a D-arginine residue of methyl arginine into position 8 resulted in practically complete loss of smooth muscle activity in the blood vessels.

Altura (1974, 1975) and Cort, Albrecht, Novakova, Mulder and Jost (1975) have carried out more extensive studies of the effects of analogues on the vasculature. In studying the effects of analogues on the cardiovascular system, most authors have followed the pressor response. This is not a very satisfactory method of analysing the action on blood vessels, since blood pressure is an expression of the haemodynamic states of different vascular beds, the degree of contraction of different types of blood vessels and the activity of the heart. Complex autonomic reflexes may further blurr the issue. Cort and his associates however pursued the regional haemodynamic effects of vasopressin analogues, whereas Altura followed the response of individual arteries, arterioles and veins.

Cort et al (1975) used the Saperstein technique of ^{86}RbCl distribution to follow the effects of LVP analogues on regional blood flow. They used various doses of each analogue and found that for LVP the threshold dose for pressor activity in the ganglion blocked rat was 10 - 25 ng/kg. At this dose there was no effect on myocardial blood flow, but there was a significant drop in gut and uterine blood flow. This would suggest that there was a definite regional difference in the affinity for vasopressin of the receptors in the vascular walls or a greater density of receptors in some areas. The observation would also suggest that the pressor activity of vasopressin may be of some physiological significance in that endogenous vasopressin may contribute to a shift of blood from viscera to skeletal muscle. The studies of Cort and his colleagues also throw light on the nature of the hormone receptor interactions. They confirmed that unaltered C-terminal amino acids are necessary for the pressor response. Thus desamino - N - methyl arginine vasopressin has virtually no pressor activity despite the fact that the C-terminal of the molecule is unchanged. N-terminal changes are also important. D-valine-lysine vasopressin is inactive, so it seems that even small differences in molecular shape prevent peptide receptor interaction. The steric requirements for receptor attachment of the C-terminal tripeptide to smooth muscle are very high. The persistent action of carba derivatives shows that, as with oxytocin, the disulphide linkage is not required to bring about smooth muscle contraction. It also appears that, by preparing carba derivatives and thereby increasing the metabolic stability of the S-S bridge, the duration of the vasoconstriction is prolonged considerably.

Prolongation of activity can also be produced by the preparation of slow release hormones such as triglycyl vasopressin (TGLVP). In view of the properties of TGLVP and carba vasopressin, Cort et al feel that they would be of value in reduction of bleeding both from the gut and the uterus, and for the induction of menstruation.

Altura (1974-1975), studying the binding of analogues to blood vessels, has thrown further light on the structural characteristics for receptor hormone interaction and intrinsic activity. He too found that the terminal amino group was important and was able to demonstrate that the phenylhydroxyl aromatic ring and basic residues in positions 2,3 and 8 were also necessary for activity in rat aortic strips, mesenteric arterioles *in vivc* and *in vitro*. This is not to say that he necessarily felt the receptors to be identical in nature. He studied the effect of a number of different analogues on the preparations and showed that the potency varied in different vessels. Despite previous reports, basicity in position 8 however is not an absolute requirement for blood vessel contraction. Studies with antagonists of AVP are needed to establish the significance of the apparent heterogeneity of vasopressin receptors in different blood vessels.

Inhibitors of Vasopressin Action

A number of synthetic analogues have been prepared which act as antagonists of vasopressin. Thus Meienhofer, Trzeciak, Dousa, Hechter, Havran, Schwartz and Walter, (1969) showed that vasopressinoic acid inhibits the antidiuretic of the naturally occurring hormone. Apart from being valuable investigative tools, antagonists could potentially be used in the treatment of patients with inappropriate vasopressin in secretion. Dyckes, Nester Ferger, De Vigneaud and Chan, (1974) investigated the properties of analogues of oxytocin and lysine vasopressin in which alterations had been made in positions 1 and 4 - namely (l - β - mercapto - β, β diethylpropionic acid, 4 - leucine - 8 lysine) vasopressin and (1 - β - mercapto - β, β - diethylpropionic acid, 4 - leucine) oxytocin. Both these analogues inhibited the oxytocic, vasopressor and avian depressor responses to neurohypophysial hormones, but did not affect antidiuretic activity. Nestor and Ferger (1975) also looked at an analogue of oxytocin substituted in position 4 - (4 phenyl alanine) oxytocin. This compound inhibited the antidiuretic response to exogenous vasopressin and in high doses caused a natriuresis.

Two agents which bind sulphydryl groups, N - ethyl maleimide and p - chloromercuribenzoate, have been shown to inhibit vasopressin-stimulated transport across the isolated toad bladder. This would suggest that these are sulphydryl groups essential for the hydro-osmotic response at or near the vasopressin receptor. In order to examine the nature of the essential sulphydryl groups Rich, Gesseellchen, Tong, Cheung and Buckner (1975) developed a method for synthesizing maleimide derivatives of oxytocin. These compounds were able to inhibit vasopressin-induced water loss from isolated toad bladders. The results further indicated that sulphydryl groups essential for the response were on the mucosal side as well as the serosal side. The authors suggested that the two compounds (1 - (N-maleolylglycyl) cysteinyl oxytocin and (1 - (N - maleoyl - 11-amino decanoyl) cysteinyl) oxytocin could be of value as affinity labelling reagents.

Summary and Conclusions

A number of studies have been performed on the conformation of vasopressin and the arrangement of the constituent amino acids has been described. Work has also continued on the structure-activity relationships with a view to gaining a greater understanding of hormone - receptor interaction. A number of analogues have also been synthesised with prolonged or enhanced biological activity. Two of these analogues have now been used in clinical practice: the first being DDAVP which has been used to treat diabetes insipidus and the second POR-8, which has been used in local anaesthetic mixtures in, for example, dentistry.

Chapter 4

ASSAY OF VASOPRESSIN

"(So the crew would protest)"That he's brought us the best a perfect and absolute blank!"

Advances in the understanding of the physiology of vasopressin have, as is the case with other hormones, been in some measure dependent on the development of a sensitive assay. In contrast to many hormones, however, a number of bioassays or functional assays were readily established. By the end of the sixties some fairly sensitive bioassays were routinely being used in studies on the factors affecting the release of the hormone. AVP has a number of biological activities upon which hormone assay is based, the main ones being the effect on the contraction of smooth muscle, especially vascular smooth muscle, and the antidiuretic action in the kidney. Action on smooth muscle has largely been used in the pressor assay in the rat (as recommended by the British Pharmacopoeia,1974) although *in vitro* preparations using rabbit rectum have been described (Gilmore and Vane, 1970). The pressor assay is relatively insensitive, so that the antidiuretic assay in the water-loaded rat anaesthetised with alcohol has been used to detect circulating levels. The assay has a lower limit of detection of about 1μU which is not sufficiently sensitive to detect circulating levels of AVP in untreated plasma.Extraction methods have therefore been developed to concentrate the hormone from plasma. These have involved chromatographic techniques as described by Weinstein, Bern and Sachs, (1960) and precipitation methods as described by Bisset, Clark, Haldar, Harris, Lewis and Rocha e Silva (1967). Chard (1975) has touched on some of the problems of vasopressin assay.

The bioassay is relatively capricious and time-consuming, so that with the advent of radioimmunoassay a number of attempts were made to adapt the technique to the estimation of AVP. Despite the considerable effort devoted to the radioimmunoassay, relatively few sensitive assays have been developed. This is largely due to the failure to produce a sufficiently sensitive antiserum.This has been achieved by a number of groups (e.g. Robertson, Klein, Roth and Gordon, 1970) although early assays were troubled with non-specificity and very high levels in plasma were reported.

Because of the problems in establishing a radioimmunoassay for vasopressin, bioassay is still extensively used and of the papers appearing during the year in which vasopressin has been estimated over 50% relied on bioassay determination.

Bioassay additionally has to be used in standardizing hormone preparations and is valuable for monitoring radioimmunoassay. Solovera (1975) has briefly reviewed bioassay techniques.

In addition to standardisation, Pituitary extracts, of course, may contain almost equal quantities of AVP and oxytocin and since Nakano (1964) reported that large doses of oxytocin caused a drop in arterial blood pressure in rats, Huang and Young (1973) investigated the influence of the vasopressor action of arginine vasopressin in the rat. They were able to show that neither injection of oxytocin given with vasopressin, in the ratio oxytocin: vasopressin of 1:1 or 1:2 nor continuous infusion of oxytocin in any way altered the pressor response to vasopressin. The presence of approximately equimolar amounts of oxytocin in pituitary extracts does not, therefore, interfere with the pressor assay for AVP.

A description of an antidiuretic assay applied to clinical situations has also appeared recently (Borner, 1975). The preparation was the water–loaded rat anaesthetised with alcohol and maintained in a constant state of hydration by placing the animal on a balance and replacing fluid as it was lost. The response parameter used in antidiuretic assay has been either urine flow (Share, 1961), urinary conductivity (Moran, Miltenberger, Shuayb and Zimmerman, 1974) or a combination of the two. Borner measured conductivity as he felt this gave a more precise assay, sensitive to 3.0 μU. When combined with an extraction method, the assay had a sensitivity of 1.0 μU/ml. The extraction method employed was a modification of the method described by Weinstein et al (1960) employing an Amberlite column. It had a mean recovery of 82 + 5% (SEM), the range being 60.6 to 95.2%. Unfortunately, lysine vasopressin (LVP) was used as the standard, which is not equipotent with AVP, (Berde and Boissonas, 1968), neither is the dose response curve parallel with that for AVP (Fabian, 1970).

Most of the techniques adopted for the extraction of plasma for bioassay are fairly tedious and cumbersome. However, Forsling (1974) described the application to bioassay of a relatively simple technique originally developed for the radioimmunoassay. Vasopressin is absorbed from acidified plasma onto a small quantity of a silicate (Spherosil X0A400), which is then washed and subsequently eluted with aqueous acetone. The eluate can then be blown down to dryness and redissolved in the appropriate diluent. The recovery with this method is 54 + 6.5% (SD, n = 25).

Radioimmunoassay

The basic requirements for a radioimmunoassay are, of course, a pure hormone preparation, a high affinity antiserum, radioactivity labelled hormone and a means of separating bound from free hormone. At present there is no standard preparation for the immunoassay of vasopressin, but a recent WHO report (1975) recommended that the use of synthetic arginine vasopressin be investigated for this purpose. As already mentioned, production of a suitable antiserum has presented considerable problems. First, a small molecular weight peptide is relatively non-immunogenic and second, arginine vasopressin is the native hormone in most species. The first problem may be overcome by conjugating the hormone to a large molecular weight protein. Thyroglobulin has been successfully used for the purpose. To overcome the second problem one might use a non-mammalian species to raise the antiserum, or a pig, in which the natural hormone is lysine vasopressin.Skowsky, Rosenbloom and Fisher (1974), on the other hand, have used lysine vasopressin to produce antisera in the rabbit. It has, however, been possible to raise antisera against arginine vasopressin in the rabbit.

Fyhrquist and Wallenius (1975) have described a method of improving antisera raised against polypeptide hormones. Rabbits used for immunisation sometimes exhibit the symptoms of deficiency of the particular hormone involved. Thus rabbits immunised with AVP do on occasions develop diabetes insipidus (Morton and Waite, 1972) and in these animals the AVP levels are markedly elevated (Forsling, unpublished observations). The sensitivity of the immunoassay could, therefore, be limited by the endogenous vasopressin which may block some of the antibody binding sites. Fyhrquist and Wallenius, therefore, reasoned that if they broke the antigen–antibody bond with a substance such as sodium iodide, they would improve the antisera. They treated antisera raised against LVP with sodium iodide, dialysed the product and then prepared dose response curves using both the treated and untreated antiserum. After iodide treatment the apparent affinity of the antiserum changed from $2.1 \times 10^{-13} M^{-1}$ to $7.1 \times 10^{-13} M^{-1}$ and the lower limit of detection of the standard curve improved ten times. It would appear therefore that this treatment unmasked high affinity binding sites on the antibody. Specificity was also increased following sodium iodide treatment. That is to say that in these studies, where antisera were raised against LVP, the sensitivity for this peptide was increased as compared with AVP. The paradoxical increase in binding of label with increasing doses of unlabelled hormone sometimes seen at low hormone concentrations was also eliminated in these experiments. Vaneckova, Barthova, Barth, Krejci and Rychlik (1975) describe a method of affinity chromatography for isolating specific antibodies raised against lysine vasopressin coupled to bovine serum albumin through the NH_2 groups. The support materials or immunosorbents used for chromatography were Sepharose 4B and Spheron P-300.

The immunosorbents were prepared by activating the solid phase using cyanogen bromide and then coupling lysine vasopressin, also through the NH_2 group. Both the immunosorbents, prepared efficiently, absorbed the antibodies to vasopressin. The antibodies could be recovered by elution with citrate buffer at pH 3.2, 6 M urea or 6 M guanidine. However, the yield was relatively poor, only 20 to 30% of the serum antibodies being absorbed.

The assays published during the year have been based on antisera raised against the conjugated hormone. Van Wimersma-Greidanus, Bohus, Hollemans and de Yong (1974), used as the antigen, AVP coupled to thyroglobulin with ethylcarbodiimide. Morton, Padfield and Forsling (1975) and Burguburu and Geelen (1974) on the other hand used albumin coupled AVP. Fukuchi, Nakajima, Takeuchi, Nishizato, Michimata (1975) have used γ-globulin coupled AVP.

Chloramine T has almost routinely been used in the iodination of AVP and this indeed is the technique used by all these groups. Van Wimersma-Greidanus et al stopped the reaction by the addition of human serum; Morton et al transferred the reaction mixture to a G25 column and then carried out separation of the reaction mixture to produce a product free from unlabelled AVP.

Separation of bound from free hormone on the whole presents no problems with small peptide hormones such as AVP as the physico-chemical properties of an octapeptide are so greatly different from the globulin-bound hormone. Probably the simplest method of separating bound from free labelled AVP is precipitation or solvent fractionation of the antibody with commonly used reagents such as ammonium sulphate, (Edwards, Chard, Kitau, Forsling and Landon, 1972). Two methods widely used in radioimmunoassay are the second antibody method, in which the antibody hormone complex is precipitated using an antibody raised in a second species, and the plasma-coated charcoal method in which the free hormone is adsorbed onto activated charcoal. Both these methods, which have been reviewed in detail elsewhere (Kirkham and Hunter, 1971), have been used in the assay of vasopressin and have been adopted by Burguburu and Geelen, Morton et al and Fressinaud, Carrol, Menard and Allegrini (1974). Another method widely used in the United States is that of Hussain, Fernando, Shapiro, Kagan and Glick (1973) using polyethylene glycol and bovine globulin to precipitate antibody bound hormone.

Radioimmunoassay has the advantage over bioassay in that it is relatively less time consuming. As already mentioned, many of the extraction methods developed for bioassay are fairly complex and, if applied to immunoassay, much of the advantage of speed would be lost. In addition the extracts produced may contain relatively large quantities of salt which would interfere with the binding of the hormone by antibody. Batchwise methods employing an adsorbant have been developed for radioimmunoassay. The general principle is the same as that in the method used by Forsling (1974). The AVP is adsorbed from the plasma onto the material, generally silicate in nature. In this way the extract contains no salt or protein. The hormone is then eluted using an organic solvent and taken to dryness, either in a rotary evaporator or under a stream of nitrogen or air. Morton et al employed the adsorbant Florisil, as did Burguburu and Geelen, in the extraction of vasopressin. The Florisil is first pretreated by washing, to remove the "fines", and then activated at 120°C for 18h. After mixing with the plasma samples, the Florisil is washed and later eluted with aqueous acetone. The mean recovery was 60 + 6.9% (range 47 - 69%) giving a lower limit of sensitivity of the assay of 2.0 pmol/1 (approx. 0.8μU/ml). Hussain et al used a method employing acetone precipitation followed by partition against ether. The acetone phase is then blown down to dryness. While all the assays described here involve an extraction step, Wagner, Maier, Herrmann and Franz (1975) have reported an immunoassay performed on unextracted serum.

Plasma Vasopressin Concentration

Basal AVP concentrations in plasma in a number of species have been reported during the year. Commonly values of around 1 - 3μU/ml have been found in all species studied. The concentrations quoted for man mainly fall within this range. Borner, using a bioassay, reports concentrations of 3.8 ± 0.3 μU/ml in normally hydrated individuals, increasing to 6.5 ± 0.55 μU/ml when the plasma is relatively hypertonic. Davies and Forsling (1975), also using bioassay, reported a concentration of 1.1 ± 0.3 μU/ml in mildly dehydrated subjects. Concentrations could increase to 15 μU/ml following syncope.

Radioimmunoassay estimates are similar to those obtained by bioassay. Morton et al found that, in healthy male subjects following an overnight fast, the mean plasma concentration was 5.3 pmol/l (approx. 2.3 μU/ml) with a range of 4.6 to 6.2 pmol/l, increasing to between 5.9 and 9.5 pmol/l following dehydration. George, Messerli, Genest, Nowaczynski, Boucher, Kuchel and Rojo-Ortego (1975) reported slightly lower levels (1.08 ± 0.14 (SEM) pg/ml or 1.00 pmol/l. These authors found that AVP shows a diurnal variation, the concentration increasing during the night by 2 pg/ml on average. More recently developed assays confirm these values. Uhlich, Weber, Groschel-Stewart and Roschlau (1975) quote early morning values of 3.4 ± 1.6 pg/ml. The resting values in normal hydrated subjects was found by Katz to be 1.8 ± 0.5 (SEM) pg/ml (personal communication) and by Thomas and Lee to be 0.57 ± 0.20 (SD) pg/ml (personal communication). Wagner et al (1975) reported higher values, 20.7 ± 8.7 μU/ml in dehydrated subjects and

Figure 4.1

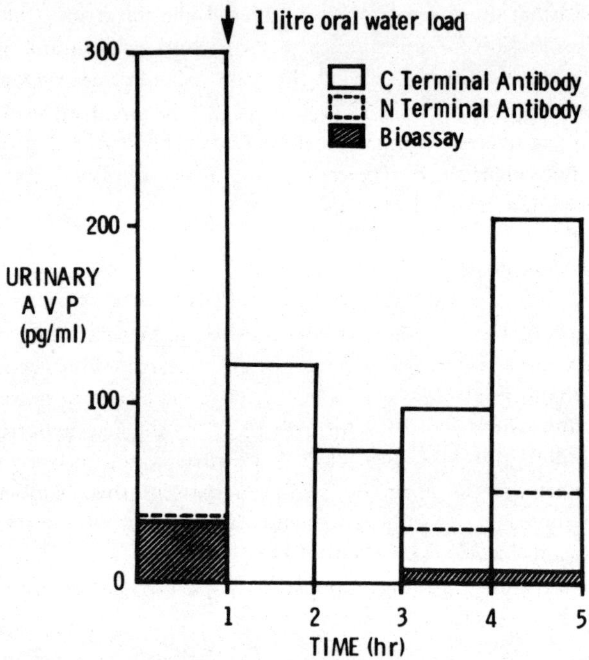

Urinary excretion of vasopressin in a control subject before and after a water load. Estimates made by bioassay and radioimmunoassay using two different antisera [Forsling, unpublished observations].

0.9 ± 7μU/ml after water load of 20ml/kg body weight.

It would seem that there is some variation in the concentrations found with radioimmunoassay. It is probable that the values obtained depend on the particular antiserum used. In reporting results of vasopressin assays therefore, care should be taken to indicate the particular antiserum used. Ideally, material measured should be further identified by checking values obtained against a biological assay. Without this type of confirmation the substance measured should strictly be called "vasopressin-like". Dissociation of antidiuretic activity and of immunological cross reactivity can and has occurred, as in the case of tumour extracts (Rees and Ratcliffe, 1974). Dissociation of activities may also occur in urine. Fig. 4.1 shows that the excretory patterns of antidiuretic activity and material measured by immunoassay are not identical.Furthermore, the levels obtained by immunoassay depend on the particular antiserum used.

Urinary Assay of Vasopressin

Because of the problems of assay of vasopressin in plasma, some workers have turned to urinary estimates of the hormone. The hormone concentration in the urine is higher than in plasma and it has been argued that because of the short half time of vasopressin in plasma, urinary AVP could give a better idea of the secretion rate. Miller and Moses developed a urinary immunoassay in 1971. Excretion of the hormone in normally hydrated man in this assay appears to be 1.0 ± 0.9 mU/h increasing to 2.74 ± 0.54 mU/h after 14h dehydration (Miller and Moses, 1972). Oyama, Kagan and Click (1971) produced a very sensitive assay and found similar values; the excretion increased to 1.2 to 6.5 mU/h after 24h dehydration.

Khokhar, Hough and Slater (1974) have applied a urinary assay for AVP to the investigation of essential hypertension. This assay, which was demonstrated to the Physiological Society (Forsling, Khokhar, Ramage and Slater 1975), is based on the method of Edwards et al (1972). In contrast to the other assays described the antisera were raised against unconjugated vasopressin. Spherosil glass beads were used as the adsorbant in the extraction method and the recovery ranged from 90% from distilled water and to 40% if urinary osmolatity was 1200 mOsm/Kg.

Fressinaud et al (1974) have also developed a radioimmunoassay for the detection of urinary vasopressin in man. Their assay, however, depends on an antiserum raised against LVP and a preparation of monoiodinated ^{125}I-LVP. Despite this fact they found identical urinary vasopressin concentrations in a parallel study using an antibody which cross-reacts more specifically with AVP. The urine was extracted using a Rexyn column eluted with 75% ethanol in water. They reported an excretion of 7.82 ± 1.56 ng/2h in dehydrated subjects which was reduced to 2.69 ± 0.4 ng/2h after a water load of 15 ml/kg and increased to 20.28 ± 1.94 ng/2h after infusion of hypertonic saline. There was a good correlation between plasma osmolality and urinary AVP, the hormone first appearing in the urine when the plasma osmolality was 275.2 mOsm/kg. On the basis of these results Fressinaud et al feel that this assay provides a valuable tool in assessing neurohypophysial function in man.

Lishajko and Anderson (1975) have developed a bioassay technique for the determination of vasopressin in the urine of goats. They used the same species, namely the goat, for the bioassay. They employed a resin column (Amberlite IRC-50, XE64) as described by Ruch (1967) for the adsorption and separation of vasopressin from urine. A modification which they introduced was to run 50% ethanol through the column before elution. This step removed interfering factors in the extract without affecting the recovery of the hormone. The assay could detect urinary vasopressin to the nearest 0.5 mU. Vasopressin was found to be excreted at 1 mU/h in the hydrated goat with the rate increasing to 8 mU/h after 48h dehydration. They estimate from these figures that the basal secretion rate of vasopressin in the water-replete animal is 5 μU/Kg/min.

Summary and Conclusions

For many years studies on vasopressin were limited through lack of a relatively simple assay. Radioimmunoassay seemed to provide the answer, but has not as yet fulfilled its promise, largely because of the want of a suitable antiserum to vasopressin. Immunisation of rabbits with vasopressin coupled to thyroglobulin appears to provide one answer to the problem. A number of assays of seemingly good specificity and fair sensitivity have been developed and it will be of interest to see how successfully they can be applied to investigations.

Chapter 5

SYNTHESIS AND SECRETION OF VASOPRESSIN

"The method employed I would gladly explain,
While I have it so clear in my head"

Largely through the efforts of Sachs (on the synthesis of vasopressin) and Douglas (on the release), a model for turnover of vasopressin in the neurohypophysis has been proposed, upon which work may be based. The studies of Sachs, depending to a large extent on observations of the incorporation of radioactive label into vasopressin, have led to the precursor theory for the synthesis of vasopressin. A precursor of the hormone is said to be synthesised on the ribosomes in the perikaryon of the hypothalamic nuclei. It is suggested that this precursor could be common to neurophysin. Once synthesised the precursor molecule(s) are packed into neurosecretory granules, probably at the Golgi apparatus. The granules are then transported, along the axons, to the posterior pituitary, either in the axonal stream or possibly along microtubules. A specialised pathway for the transport of neurosecretory vesicles has been proposed, since the estimated rate of axonal transport of 1 - 4mm/h (Norstrom and Sjostrand, 1971; Pickering and Jones, 1971), is ten times greater than normally observed for axoplasmic flow. Active vasopressin is said to be formed as the granules descend to the neural lobe. Vasopressin is then released from the neurohypophysis in association with neurophysin (Forsling, Martin, Sturdy & Burton, 1973) in response to propagated action potentials, which result in ion influx, depolarisation and probably exocytosis. There is considerable evidence to suggest that this process, termed stimulus-secretion coupling, is calcium dependent. Extensive speculation and discussion have surrounded the possible mechanisms of release, but there is increasing evidence to support the concept of exocytosis, which has been reviewed by Douglas (1974) who does, however, admit to some possible bias. Much of this evidence has been reviewed by Vollrath (1974).

Synthesis of Vasopressin

Little new work has appeared during the year on the synthesis of vasopressin, but two new preparations have been developed, as mentioned in chapter 2, which may provide useful tools for investigating this topic. Pearson, Shainberg, Osinchak and Sachs (1975) describe a preparation in organ culture of guinea pig hypothalamus and neurohypophysis which could be maintained for up to three weeks. Although synthesis of RNA was impaired initially after four to five days it was restored to normal as was protein synthesis. This recovery of protein metabolism and RNA synthesis was paralleled by similar biosynthetic activity of vasopressin. In the other preparation a clone of mouse hypothalamic neurosecretory cells was established (De Vitry, Camier, Czernichow, Benda, Cohen and Tixier-Vidal, 1974). These cells too, were capable of incorporating ^{35}S-label into peptides with the same chemical and immunochemical characteristics as vasopressin and neurophysin. Exploitation of these techniques must certainly throw fresh light on the mode of synthesis. An example of this is seen in the foetal studies described in chapter 15.

Storage and Release of Vasopressin

Vasopressin exists as a biologically active peptide in the neurohypophysis, although probably initially produced as the precursor molecule. Supporting evidence that this conversion occurs as the neurosecretory granules travel down the hypothalamus has been provided by Dyball and Henry (1975). They followed the changes in vasopressin and milk-ejecting activities in the supraoptic region in the hypothalamus of rats at various intervals after hypophysectomy. An earlier observation, that there was an increase in the number of neurosecretory granules of the supraoptic nucleus after hypophysectomy, correlates with the results of these studies where there was an increase in biological activity in extracts of that nucleus after hypophysectomy. Increase of neurosecretory material thus represents stored hormone. This stored material is unable to descend to the pituitary so that maturation occurs in the hypothalamus. Thus the increase in measured biological activity supports the hypothesis that an initial inactive precursor molecule is formed which subsequently gives rise to the active peptide. There was a relatively greater increase in milk-ejecting activity which gave rise to speculation that the final maturation of oxytocin might occur more slowly than vasopressin, since if this were the case there would have been relatively more inactive oxytocin present originally.

Another manoeuvre which alters the neurohypophysial hormone content of hypothalamic nuclei and tract is saline dehydration. Grainger and Sloper (1974) have used this stimulus to investigate the mechanisms by which secretory material is transported along the tractus hypophysis. There is increased turnover of hormones in animals given hypertonic saline to drink and this is associated with a conspicuous increase in the number of microtubules. An even greater increase as compared with normal animals, was seen in animals with congenital diabetes insipidus. An increase in the turnover of neurohypophysial hormones would be consistent with an increase in microtubules if the latter are involved in the transport mechanisms. Flament-Durand and Dustin (1974) have provided evidence that this is the case. In their experiments colchicine was shown to interrupt the flow of neurosecretory granules in the paraventricular neurones. Synthesis of protein was not affected.

Krisch (1974) has carried out an electron microscope study on the effect of dehydration on the morphology of the hypothalamo-hypophysial tract. After 48h water deprivation, changes were manifest in both the supra-optic and paraventricular nuclei. Especially notable was the fact that the diameter of the neurosecretory granules in the supraoptic nucleus was less than those in the pituitary. It was, therefore, suggested that in stress, the hormone is packed into smaller granules, if packed at all.

Once in the posterior lobe some of the hormone is said to be in a readily releasable form. Pickering, Jones and Burford (1974) summarised their recent studies on biochemistry of hypothalamo-neurohypophysial neurones and present new evidence for a readily releasable pool. They followed the incorporation and distribution of ^{35}S labels using electron microscope autoradiography. The label appeared first at the fine nerve endings and then moved back into the larger nerve endings. It would appear therefore that if newly synthesised material is not released it is stored for release in severe conditions if needed.

Dreifuss, Nordman, Akert, Sandri and Moor (1974) have provided fresh evidence to show that hormone is released by exocytosis. They stimulated hormone release from isolated rat neurohypophyses by electrical stimulation or by exposure to high potassium concentration, to lanthanum or to cold. They used the technique of freeze fracture to demonstrate changes within membranes of stimulated neurosecretory nerve terminals. They found that the plasma membrane showed numerous modulations which would be unnecessary if release occurred by simple diffusion. These authors rather believe that the changes reflect underlying exocytosis. Dempsey, Bullivant and Watkins (1974) have applied the same technique to the study of membranes of the neurohypophysis removed from rats in various states of dehydration. During exocytosis the membrane of the secretory granule attaches itself to the cell membrane and the two fuse. There should be evidence of this in freeze fracture studies; "holes" should be formed where the membranes fuse and broken-off "necks". Evidence of these structures was found in normal rats and the numbers increased after 2 days dehydration. Douglas (1974) has suggested that this exocytosis is due to calcium ions.

Preparations of undamaged pre-synaptic nerve endings have been used to study the underlying events in neurotransmission (deBelleroche and Bradford, 1975). Bennet and Edwardson (1975) have prepared neurosecretory nerve endings or synaptosomes from the hypothalamus of the sheep and the rat. They were found to contain corticotrophin releasing factor, prolactin-release inhibiting factor and vasopressin and appeared to retain much of their morphological and functional integrity when incubated *in vitro*. Thus electrical stimulation or application of potassium (55mmol/l) resulted in a calcium-dependent secretion of the various factors from the synaptosomes. These preparations would seem to provide an additional valuable tool for studying neurosecretion.

Role of Calcium in Vasopressin Release

The evidence that calcium influx is central in stimulus - secretion coupling is not as strong for neurohypophysial cells as chromaffin cells. However, many parallels exist between secretion from chromaffin cells and the neurohypophysis. Impetus has, therefore, been lent to the search for evidence that calcium is a secretogogue in the posterior pituitary. To demonstrate a role for calcium it is necessary to show that elevation of calcium mimics the response. Depending on the situation, this elevation may be produced by microinjection, by ionophores, by sodium replacement or ouabain. If the calcium involved in the response is of extracellular origin, it should be possible to demonstrate that the response is associated with calcium efflux, that it is proportional to the calcium ion concentration and that it may be blocked by calcium inhibitors. If the calcium is of intracellular origin, none of these criteria apply, but the response should be accompanied by calcium efflux. Using these criteria, Thorn and his colleagues have been able to establish that calcium is an essential link in the stimulus-secretion coupling, (Thorn 1974, 1975).

Ionophores, drugs which facilitate the transport of cations across biological membranes, have been applied to the problem. An antibiotic ionophore A-23187 specifically facilitating transmembrane-flux of divalent cations was described by Reed and Lardy in 1972. Russell, Hansen and Thorn (1974) have investigated the effect of this agent on a preparation routinely used by Thorn in the investigation of vasopressin secretion -- namely isolated hemilobes of rat neurohypophysis. If A-23187 was incubated with the neural lobes in a calcium-free medium, then there was an increase in the secretion of vasopressin when calcium was added to the medium. Addition of the ionophore to the bathing medium also caused an increased efflux of pre-loaded $^{45}Ca^{++}$ which probably resulted from increased calcium exchange. These results were taken to indicate that the ionophore elevated intracellular calcium by an increase in inward transport and that this increase resulted in stimulation of vasopressin release.

Thorn, Russell and Robinson (1975) were able to confirm that the site of action of the ionophore is at the plasma membrane by using the D-600. This ionophore which is thought to act solely on the calcium channels of the membrane reduced the effect of A-23187 on vasopressin release.

Russell et al made the alternative suggestion that the increased calcium efflux resulted from release of calcium from intracellular structures. This second explanation is favoured by Nordman and Currell (1975). They argued that, since calcium efflux persisted in the absence of external calcium, sodium and magnesium ions, it was most likely that the ionophore they used - X-537A - raised the intracellular level of calcium directly. This belief was strengthened by the fact that X537A increases the efflux of calcium ions from isolated brain mitochondria. Nevertheless these data corroborate the essential role of the concentration of intracellular calcium ions in stimulus-secretion coupling.Thorn et al (1975) using the ionophore D-600 also obtained evidence for intracellular nature of X 537A action.

The sulphydryl reagent n-ethyl maleimide appears to enhance vasopressin release through a similar effect on accumulation of free Ca ions in the neurosecretory terminals (Russell, Warberg and Thorn, 1974). Incubations of preparations of rat neurohypophyses with NEM resulted in prolonged elevation of vasopressin release, correlated with efflux of the $^{45}Ca^{++}$ with which the tissue had been previously labelled. NEM probably reduced the binding of calcium to intracellular membranes since thiol agents are known to act in this way in other systems. In order for the vasopressin-releasing system to work efficiently there must be an efficient binding of calcium to intracellular membranes in order that excess calcium may be rapidly removed after stimulation.

Further results stressing the importance of both extracellular and intracellular calcium in the release of vasopressin have come from the laboratories of Thorn (Muller, Thorn and Torp-Pedersen 1975). It was noted that after prolonged stimulation of rat neurohypophysis *in vitro* with 56mM potassium in the absence of calcium, late addition of this latter ion augmented vasopressin secretion. Elevated secretion also accompanied the removal of sodium provided that calcium ions were present. These findings would appear to argue against depletion of a readily releasable pool as a reason for the decline of secretion and are more consistent with inactivation of one of the steps involved.

Russell and Thorn (1974) also investigated the role of calcium in vasopressin release from isolated pituitaries following electrical stimulation. This type of stimulation led to a 5–8 fold increase in vasopressin release over basal levels which was calcium dependent. Only very small quantities of calcium must be involved in the response as there was no demonstrable increase in the uptake of ^{45}Ca into slices of posterior lobe tissue.

Nordman (1975) too, has demonstrated a possible relationship between calcium entry and vasopressin release from isolated rat neurohypophyses. On prolonged exposure (120 mins) to a high potassium concentration of 56mmol/l hormone release, although at first stimulated, is not maintained. This drop in hormone output is paralleled by a fall in ^{45}Ca uptake. It seems likely that reduced hormone secretion results from inactivation of calcium entry.

The finding of Dreifuss, Grau and Nordmann (1975), that cobalt, manganese and D-600 reduce both calcium uptake and hormone secretion from the isolated rat neurohypophysis in a dose-dependent way, suggests that calcium entry upon stimulation is via membrane channels similar to those postulated for the axon terminal in the squid (Katz and Miledi, 1967). The further evidence that tetrodotoxin, in concentrations which abolished the compound action potential, affected neither potassium-stimulated hormone release nor the accompanying ^{45}Ca uptake, also indicates that calcium entry is not via "sodium channels".

In the face of such evidence there is no gainsaying the central role of calcium in stimulus-secretion couplings in the neurohypophysis. However, as already mentioned, for calcium to trigger secretion by increasing intracellular free calcium, it has normally to be maintained below a certain critical level in quiescent conditions. This could be achieved by active extrusion of calcium and/or by binding to intracellular components. In support of this second suggestion, Russell and Thorn (1975) have provided evidence for the accumulation of calcium by microsomal and mitochondrial fractions, in the presence of ATP, by far the greater uptake being onto the microsomal fraction. The uptake which was accompanied by liberation of inorganic phosphate was both temperature and pH dependent and also required magnesium ions. The presence of NEM inhibited both calcium uptake and phosphate liberation from the microsomal fraction to the same extent. Further, if incubation of this fraction was carried out in a calcium free medium, phosphate release increased if calcium was added. It appears, therefore, that the magnesium-calcium-activated ATPase is associated with calcium uptake into the microsomal fraction of bovine neurohypophysis and this could, in part, aid in the maintainance of a low resting intracellular calcium concentration.

Poisner and Hong (1974) showed that this ATP-activated uptake of calcium into cell fractions was blocked by low temperature. Instead there was release of calcium from the isolated neurohypophysis. They suggested therefore that cold-induced release of AVP could be due to an increase in cytoplasmic calcium which stimulates the normal pathways for release. They also studied release of vasopressin from the neurohypophysis neurosecretory granules and suggest that these preparations could be useful for studying the mechanisms underlying storage and release of the hormone.

Subsequent studies on the neurosecretory granules revealed a possible method of cold-induced vasopressin, (Hong and Poisner, 1974). Bovine neurohypophyses were used in the preparation of neurosecretory granules both at 25°C or 0°C. The granules prepared at 25°C contained substantially greater quantities of vasopressor activity but were more susceptible to lysis by cold temperature and tonicity than granules prepared at 0°C; it seems, therefore, that the most freely releasable material was lost in the preparation of granules at 0°C. The change underlying the observations seen at room temperature was an initial phase transition of the lipids of the granule membranes which resulted in increasing the permeability to various ions. Osmotic passage of water into the granules then caused them to swell and finally lyse, liberating soluble constituents into the medium. In evidence of this proposal they show that exposure to hypertonic solution enhances cold-induced vasopressin release from granules prepared at room temperature and that this can be inhibited by sucrose. Lanthanum methyl sulphate which limits ion penetration of the membrane and lauryl alcohol, which probably stabilizes the membrane, were effective in inhibiting the loss of vasopressin from neurosecretory granules. Hong and Poisner also point out as a result of these studies, that it is important to control temperature in studying the release of vasopressin, using *in vitro* preparations.

Summary and Conclusions

Little new information has appeared during the year on the synthesis of vasopressin but preparations of the neurohypophysial system in culture have been described which should allow valuable additional approaches to the problem. The time–sequence of events should thus be easily followed. As far as the release of the hormone is concerned, the main body of work appearing has been devoted to consolidating a central role for calcium. Thorn has solidly defended the central role of calcium in the release of vasopressin and has shown that ionophores and NEM affect both intracellular calcium and vasopressin release. He feels that only a 'trigger pulse' of calcium may be required since the evidence of a net uptake of calcium on stimulation is weak in many situations . It has been further proposed that intracellular calcium concentration is maintained by ATP dependent uptake onto microsomal membranes.

Chapter 6

PATHWAYS AND TRANSMITTERS IN VASOPRESSIN RELEASE

"Then subtract Seventeen, and the answer must be
Exactly and perfectly true"

A number of studies have been performed on the central pathways involved in neurohypophysial hormone release, especially oxytocin release. This is perhaps the easier of the two hormones to study, as the milk ejection response is a good marker for the release of oxytocin, being fairly specific for oxytocin and relatively easy to follow. Besides the osmotic control of vasopressin, many other factors appear to modify vasopressin release. It appears that much of this afferent information travels in spinothalamic tracts and vagus. It is likely that the information passes along extralemniscal tracts in the central tegmentum. Before entering the hypothalamus, the main pathways probably relay in the thalamus. However, there is evidence that the periventricular system and the median forebrain bundles are involved.

The final common pathway is the neurosecretory cell itself. Both excitatory and inhibitory inputs supply the cells of the supraoptic and paraventricular nuclei, but it is not clear which neurotransmitters are involved. Shute and Lewis (1966) have demonstrated that cholinergic and adrenergic pathways are probably involved. Studies have been performed in the rat, in which activity was measured in the cells of both nuclei following microiontophoretic injections of putative transmitters onto the cell bodies. From such work it appears that noradrenaline is inhibitory (Moss, Dyball and Cross, 1971) and acetyl choline excitatory (Dreifuss and Kelly, 1972), the effect involving nicotinic receptors. However, Milton and Paterson (1971) have shown that, in the cat, microinjections of noradrenaline into the supraoptic nucleus stimulate vasopressin release, and Barker, Crayton and Nicoll (1971) have reported, again in the cat, that antidromically identified cells were inhibited by acetyl choline. Much of this evidence has been received by Cross (Cross, 1974; Cross and Dyball, 1974).

The Central Nervous System and Vasopressin Release

Hata and Miura (1974) have provided evidence to suggest that vasopressin release is modulated by the fastigial nucleus. Carotid occlusion is said to produce increased vasopressin release by effects on baroreceptor and chemoreceptor activity (see Chapter 9). These workers suggest that stimulation of the fastigial nucleus can attenuate this response, so that, for example, vasopressin release on changing from a recumbent to an upright posture would be reduced. They used bioassay to measure vasopressin concentration in the plasma of cats before and during carotid occlusion and then, with carotid occlusion maintained, during stimulation of the cerebellar fastigial nucleus (fastigial pressor area). The animals had a fairly high control vasopressin concentration in plasma, with a mean of 60.2 μU/m1. This value rose by a mean of 135.4 μU/m1 during carotid occlusion, but fell by 82.2 μU/m1 when the fastigial nucleus was stimulated. Cardiovascular responses to carotid occlusion were enhanced by fastigial nucleus stimulation. These differences in effect could be due to the fact that different groups of neurones are involved in the cardiovascular response. It appears that cerebellar modulation of vasopressin release occurs at the level of the lower brain stem which receives projections from the carotid sinus nerve and outflow from the fastigial pressor area.

Thomas (1975) has investigated the effect on vasopressin metabolism of stimulating the amygdala at various frequencies. He monitored release from the cut pituitary stalk and the intact pituitary gland. Electrical stimulation was performed at rates of 4 and 36 cps. It was found that antidiuretic material was released in response to high frequency stimulation of the amygdala medial nucleus.

Drugs Affecting Vasopressin Release

Several investigations have been performed on the effect of drugs on vasopressin secretion, many of them with the aim of determining the putative neurotransmitters involved. Several different types of preparation have been used, but it is difficult to compare the results of the various studies.The isolated pituitary, for example, comprises only cut nerve terminals and hence might be expected to behave differently from an intact organ. Similarly, the method of administering drugs to an intact animal, be it intravenously, intraventricularly, or iontophoretically, will affect the response.

It is generally taken that acetyl choline stimulates release of vasopressin and the investigations published during the year tend to confirm this. Marks, Sakai, George, and Koestner (1974) have developed a new technique for studying neuroendocrine systems. The tissue under investigation, in this case from the supraoptic nucleus of neonatal puppies, is isolated and maintained in organ culture for two to three weeks. The explant is then transferred to a small superfusion chamber and cell membrane potentials and action potentials recorded. This technique has been used to investigate changes in the activity of cells following the application of various drugs, in order to obtain information on the receptor mechanisms in neuroendocrine systems. The resting membrane potential of cells taken from the supraoptic nucleus and kept in organ culture was - 36 mV and the firing rate less than one per second. After they had been exposed to acetyl choline in a concentration of 10^{-7} to 10^{-5}M for one minute, the rate of firing increased to nearly 10 spikes/sec. Dihydro-beta erythroidine, a drug which blocks nicotine receptors, blocked the response but atropine, which blocks muscarinic receptors, increased the activity of the cell after acetyl choline (Sakai, Marks, George and Koestner, 1974). The results indicate the presence of stimulatory nicotinic receptors and inhibitory muscarinic receptors on the cells of the supraoptic nucleus. Kilbinger, Lohnes and Muscholl (1975), on the other hand, could find no evidence of nicotinic or muscarinic receptors in isolated rat neurohypophyses (i.e. in secretory terminal fibres). They found that acetyl choline affected neither the "resting" vasopressin release, nor potassium stimulated release.

Bridges, Hillhouse and Jones (1975) have observed the release of both vasopressin and oxytocin from rat hypothalami *in vitro*. This hypothalamic preparation comprises the supraoptic nucleus, paraventricular nucleus, median eminence and proximal pituitary stalk. Acetyl choline produced a graded increase in vasopressin secretion over the range 6.5 x 10^{-12}M to 6.5 x 10^{-10}M.

Kuhn (1974) in a series of *in vitro* studies has provided evidence of a role for muscarinic receptors. Acetyl choline injections into the third ventricle of anaesthetised rats with stereotaxically implanted needles produced a fall in urine flow and an increase in urinary electrolyte concentration. This response, which was taken as indicative of vasopressin release, was blocked by atropine and could not be mimicked by nicotine. Ruoff, Gosbee and Lederis (1974) have also taken urine flow in the anaesthetised rat as an index of vasopressin release. They perfused the neural lobe *in vivo* and found, in contrast to the neural lobe *in vitro*, acetyl choline in doses of 10 - 100 ng stimulated vasopressin release. Carbachol (5 - 20 ng) was also stimulatory. Vandeputte-Van Messon and Peeters (1974) have studied the effect on water diuresis in conscious goats of various cholinergic drugs. They found that, although acetyl choline or eserine alone have little effect, when injected together produced inhibition of a water diuresis which could be blocked by atropine. This result adds further support to the concept of a muscarinic receptor in vasopressin release.

Most of these studies on cholinergic drugs were carried out in parallel with investigations on adrenergic drugs. Thus, Marks et al (1974) studied the effects of noradrenaline and isoprenaline on the cultured cells of the supraoptic nucleus. These adrenergic agents had no effect on the 'resting' but inhibited the spike activity produced by nicotine. This effect could be reversed by propranolol.

Ruoff, et al (1974) also investigated the effect of the monoamines noradrenaline and dopamine, and found that they had no effect when applied to the rat neural lobe *in vivo*. In contrast, Kuhn (1974) found that noradrenaline, when injected into the third ventricle of hydrated, anaesthetised rats, produced an antidiuresis which could be blocked by phentolamine. These studies would indicate that synapses of α-adrenergic origin exist. Stutinsky (1974) has come to the same conclusion in experiments employing stereotaxic drug injections into the supraoptic and paraventricular nuclei of rats. He found that L-dopa and noradrenaline (2 μg) caused vasopressin release as indicated by an increase in blood pressure and an antidiuresis in the experimental animals. This antidiuretic effect was not seen after treatment with α blockers.

Bridges et al (1975) found that dopamine stimulated vasopressin release, both from isolated hypothalamic preparations and *in vivo*. Injections of dopamine of 2 -- 30 μg into the lateral cerebral ventricle produced antidiuresis and milk ejection in an anaesthetised rat. This effect was blocked by haloperidol given intravenously or into the cerebral ventricle. Vandeputte-Van Messon and Peeters (1974) also found that noradrenaline given intraventricularly to conscious goats produced an antidiuresis, which did not occur after treatment with phentolamine.

Another group of substances whose effect on vasopressin release has been studied are the prostaglandins. Uhlich, Haselbeck and Weber (1975) have treated isolated rat neurohypophyses with prostaglandin E_2 (PGE_2), which is present in the hypothalamus and PGA_2, which may be regarded as a circulating hormone. They found that both prostaglandins in a concentration of 10^{-5}M stimulated vasopressin release. Ruoff et al (1974) found that PGE_1 and $PGF_{2\alpha}$ at a lower concentration of 10^{-7}M had no effect on vasopressn release from the isolated neural lobe *in vitro*. However, *in vivo* application of PGE_1 was found to stimulate vasopressin release.

There is some evidence in mammals that vasopressin can inhibit its own release (see Chapter 8). Barker, Ifshin and Gainer (1975) have studied the effects of vasopressin and some analogues on the neurosecretory cells of molluscan preparations. They found that these peptides produced long-lasting changes in the properties of the membranes of these cells. These changes manifested themselves in the production of .bursting pacemaker potential activity which would result in an increase in secretion rather than a fall.

Angiotensin and Vasopressin Release

The suggestion that angiotensin II may affect vasopressin release has been widely quoted, although there is little direct evidence that angiotensin II stimulates vasopressin release by a central mechanism. The possibility of an interaction between vasopressin and the renin system is obviously important and further investigations could lead to a better understanding of the role of angiotensin in fluid and electrolyte balance. Gagnon and his co-workers have made a series of studies on the effects of angiotensin II on vasopressin output from isolated rat neurohypophyses *in vitro*. Gagnon, Cousineau, and Boucher (1973) showed that angiotensin II was capable of stimulating vasopressin release in this system. Stimulation only occurred if at least 0.5 mM calcium was present in the incubation medium (Gagnon, Sirois and Boucher, 1975). The response was fairly rapid, release occurring within 2.5 min of the application of angiotensin II (10^{-9} M) with a maximum at 10 min. Gagnon et al (1975) also provided evidence that cyclic AMP (cAMP) could be an intermediate in this effect. Angiotensin II produced an increase in cAMP in the neural lobe after 5 min. Theophylline also elevated vasopressin output. In an attempt to characterise the neurohypophyseal receptors for angiotensin II, Gagnon, Sirois and Park (1975) have looked at the effect on vasopressin release of angiotensin I and several analogues of angiotensin II. The decapeptide had a stimulatory effect on the neurohypophysis but there was evidence that it acted through angiotensin II. It was found that several octapeptides related to angiotensin II stimulated vasopressin release, although a longer interaction period was required if the peptide was modified in position 1. Ruoff et al (1974) using the same incubation medium as Gagnon et al, one containing 2.8 mM calcium, found that 10^{-7} M angiotensin II did not stimulate vasopressin release *in vitro*. On the contrary, it decreased output. They made the same observation *in vivo*.

Keil, Summy-Long and Severs (1975) introduced angiotensin II (0 - 100 ng) into the ventricular CSF of conscious rats and found a dose dependent release of vasopressin. The hormone estimates were carried out on trunk blood, using a sensitive radioimmunoassay. They found a resting vasopressin concentration of 2.8 ± 0.7 (SEM) pg/ml (approx 1.0 μU/ml) which rose to 25.0 ± 5.0 pg/ml when 100 ng angiotensin II were injected centrally. There is thus some disagreement as to the possible function of angiotensin II on vasopressin release, but the discrepant observations may well result from the different techniques and site of application of the peptide in the different studies.

Morphine and Vasopressin Release

It was observed many years ago that morphine could stimulate vasopressin release (DeBodo, 1944). An understanding of the mechanisms involved would be valuable in forming a picture of the central mechanisms of vasopressin release. Such knowledge could also be of value in that morphine blocking agents could well be used to reduce inappropriate vasopressin secretion. Hayward (1974) has studied the effects of morphine on vasopressin release in chronically–prepared, unanaesthetised monkeys. Low doses of morphine (1 mg/kg) produced inhibitory effects including a water diuresis. In higher doses, morphine produced excitation and caused an antidiuresis. High doses (greater than 10 mg/kg) blocked the antidiuretic effects of amygdala stimulation, although other behavioural responses persisted. Thus, in addition to being an area possibly important for vasopressin release (as described above), the amygdala may be important in the actions of morphine on motivated behaviour and vasopressin release.

Release of Transmitters from the Posterior Pituitary

Gamma amino butyric acid (GABA), thought to be a neurotransmitter in a number of pathways, is found in the posterior pituitary (Beart, Kelley and Schon, 1974). Furthermore, the pituicyte glial cells have an uptake for GABA. This raises the question of whether GABA could in any way affect neurosecretion in the posterior pituitary. Minchin and Nordmann (1975) have compared the release of preloaded [^{3}H] GABA from the isolated posterior pituitary of the rat with that of neurophysin. Electrical stimulation of the pituitary stalk of single posterior pituitary glands produced parallel increases in neurophysin release and the efflux of [^{3}H] GABA. One could therefore speculate that release of GABA from the pituicytes might form a negative feedback loop in the control of vasopressin secretion.

Traczyk (1974) followed the release of substance P and vasopressin from in situ preparations of the posterior pituitary. He used bioassay techniques to identify the two substances. He felt that the possible negative correlation between release of substance P and vasopressin should be investigated, as it could throw more light on vasopressin secretion.

Summary and Conclusions

There is some disagreement as to the nature of the putative neurotransmitters involved in vasopressin release. It appears that acetyl choline is excitatory and that both nicotinic and muscarinic receptors could be involved. The role of noradrenaline is less clear-cut, this amine being stimulatory in some preparations and inhibitory in others. It also appears that dopamine may play a role.

Chapter 7

NEUROPHYSINS

"You may seek it with thimbles - and seek it with care;
You may hunt it with forks and hope;"

It is only relatively recently in the history of the neurohypophysis that neurophysin has been discovered (Acher and Fromageot, 1957). It was originally believed that the active principle of the neurohypophysis was a protein with a molecular weight of 20 - 30,000 dalton. Van Dyke and his colleagues isolated this protein from bovine pituitary glands - hence the name "Van Dyke protein". It had however been suggested, as long ago as 1919, that there were a number of active substances in the gland (Dudley, 1919). A debate ensued but this suggestion was finally proved valid by Du Vigneaud (1953). As described in Chapter 5, neurophysin is synthesised together with vasopressin and oxytocin and its principle function is thought to be a carrier for the hormones, although other actions have been suggested. Neurophysins have been isolated from several species but those that have been best characterised are those from the cow and the pig. They are peptides with a molecular weight of 9 - 10,000 dalton and rich in disulphide groups. In most species neurophysin is not a single protein but a series of related proteins. This led to some problems with nomenclature as different groups gave the various neurophysins different names. Breslow (1975a) has attempted to collate these various names.

Neurophysin is located in the neurosecretory granules with the hormones and it has been suggested that there is one neurophysin for each neurohypophysial hormone. Lysine vasopressin has been found to be associated with porcine neurophysin I and oxytocin with neurophysin II. The "one neurophysin - one hormone" story is not entirely consistent as three neurophysins are found in several species and only one in the guinea pig. The amino acid sequence of the various neurophysins so far purified is very similar and it has also been noted that there is duplication of amino acid sequence within the polypeptide chain. This would suggest that there might be two binding sites per neurophysin molecule, but not all the experimental evidence supports this suggestion. Many studies have been performed on the amino sequences important for hormone - neurophysin interaction. This work has been discussed in full detail by Breslow (1975a). An important finding to emerge is that those features of the hormone necessary for biological activity are not the same as those required for binding to neurophysin.

Neurophysin is released into the circulation with the neurohypophysial hormones, but does not appear to bind them in plasma. It was hoped, since neurophysin was easier to measure in the circulation, that it could be used as a marker of posterior pituitary function but this has not generally proved to be the case. The kidneys are probably the main site of clearance for neurophysin. Much of the history of neurophysin has been summarised by Hope (Hope, 1975; Hope and Pickup, 1974). A number of papers concerning neurophysin have appeared during the year but only those directly involving vasopressin will be considered here. For a full review of the subject the reader is referred to the Symposium on Neurophysin Proteins held in New York in 1974 and reported in the Annals of the New York Academy of Sciences (1975).

Hormone Neurophysin Binding

At the meeting mentioned above time was spent discussing hormone-neurophysin binding (see e.g. Chaiken, Randolph and Taylor, 1975; Hruby. Spatola, Glasel and McKelvy, 1975; Cutnell, Glasel and Hruby, 1975; Pliska 1975). Breslow (1975b) summarised much of the available knowledge. As far as the hormone is concerned, the important residues for binding appear to be at positions 1 to 3, the γ - amino group of cysteine in position 1 and an aromatic residue in position 2 being particularly important. There appears to be no functional specificity of neurophysin binding to the neurohypophysial hormones (Cort, Sedlakova, Kluh and Mulder, 1975). With regard to groups in neurophysin which could participate in binding, strong evidence has been produced for the involvement of tyrosine 49. This possibility was first suggested by Furth and Hope (1970), who showed that in the nitrated protein, the tyrosine 49 microenvironment is perturbed on hormone binding. There is strong evidence for the involvement of a side-chain carboxyl group and the studies of Walter and Hoffman (1973) suggest a role for glutamic acid 3l or aspartic acid 30 of bovine neurophysin II.

While Breslow and her colleagues have suggested that the hormone binds to neurophysin on a 1:1 basis, Cohen, Camier, Wolff, Alazard, Cohen and Griffin (1975) have pointed out that under certain conditions neurophysin can bind two vasopressin molecules. They also take issue with the suggestion that there may be identity in the reaction of oxytocin and vasopressin with neurophysin. Wolff, Alazard, Camier, Griffin and Cohen (1975) have extended their studies on the possible role of tyrosine 49 in hormone-neurophysin interaction. They prepared nitro derivatives of bovine neurophysins I and II and investigated the participation of tyrosine 49 using equilibrium dialysis and ultra-violet spectroscopy. The nitrated protein bound only one molecule of 8-lysine vasopressin as opposed to the natural protein which bound two molecules. The changes which were seen in the wave length absorption maxima of nitro-tyrosine 49 provided evidence that the micro environment of this residue changes from being less to more polar. The solvent perturbation studies led these workers to conclude that the tyrosine 49 residue is unmasked by the conformational changes which occur upon complex formation.

Sedlakova, Kluh, Barth and Jost (1974), investigated the contribution to binding of the residues in the hormone, using a group of synthetic analogues. The factors they investigated were the size of the side chain of the amino acid in position 2, the contribution of the disulphide bond and the role of the linear tripeptide tail. They used gelfiltration on a Sephadex G-25 column to follow the hormone binding. All the analogues investigated could bind to neurophysin, which does raise again the specificity of the reaction. Sedlakova et al (1974) suggest that neurophysin may also bind fragments of the hormone formed during metabolic inactivation.

Most of these studies have relied on preparations of neurophysin made from acetone powder. Recently studies of Meyer–Grass and Pliska (1974), throw some doubt on the validity of using such material. They studied extracts of bovine neurosecretory granules and suggested that the "native" neurophysin may be a lipoprotein. They also indicate (Pliska, Meyer–Grass and Sunde, 1974) that this "native" neurophysin has a higher association constant for binding of vasopressin than does the material prepared in the usual way. If this is the case, the role of neurophysin as a physiological binder may have to be re-evaluated. Pliska and Meyer–Grass (1975) report low binding capacities for the material from the neurosecretory granules. This could result from molecular aggregation of neurophysin. Perhaps in the neurosecretory granules *in vivo* neurophysin exists in a precisely organised manner.

Synthesis and Release of Neurophysin

Synthesis of neurophysin has been considered in Chapter 5 and the neurophysin containing pathways have been described in Chapter 2. A number of papers have appeared which are more concerned with the turnover of the carrier protein than the hormone. Norstrom (1974, 1975) and Pickering, Jones, Burford, McPherson, Swann, Heap and Morris (1975) have summarised much of their work on the axonal transport and turnover of neurophysin proteins in the rat. Both groups of workers were able to demonstrate incorporation of ^{35}S cysteine into neurophysin after intracisternal or local injection into the supraoptic nucleus. Maximum labelling was found in the pituitary after about 12 h. This radio-activity labelled material had a half life of approximately ten days in the rat pituitary. Pickering et al (1975) found evidence of only a single rate of axonal transport whereas Norstrom (1975) believes that there is a slowly transported fraction and a more rapidly transported fraction. Both authors found evidence for a heterogeneous pool of neurophysin proteins, possibly representing an intragranular and an extragranular pool of neurophysin or a spatial distribution of granules within the nerve endings.

When the neurohypophysial system is stimulated, as for example, by haemorrhage or dehydration, there is an increase in the rate of turnover of neurophysin. The transport rate of the protein is unaffected but greater amounts of material are transported per unit time. In order to investigate the mechanism of transport, Norstrom (1975) studied the effect of local anaesthetics on the rapid axonal transport of neurophysin. Following a subarachnoid injection of tetracaine or chlorpromazine, there was a blockage of axonal transport, but no observable change in the neurotubules. This observation contrasts with that of Grainger and Sloper (1974) (see Chapter 5). Norstrom also demonstrated that glycoproteins are involved in the secretory processes in the neurohypophysis. Thorn, Russell and Vilhardt (1975) have also suggested that a hexosamine present in the secretory granule membranes and probably combined with lipoprotein could play a part in hormone turnover. The hexosamine could bind calcium but whether or not it is involved in the hormone-neurophysin interaction is not clear.

Much of the work performed on the release of the contents of the neurosecretory granules has been summarised by Dreifuss (1975) with especial reference to neurophysins. McKelvy (1975), also considering transport and release of neurophysins, has postulated a role for cyclic nucleotides. He has studied protein kinase activity associated with neurosecretory granules isolated from bovine and guinea pig neural lobes. He was able to demonstrate the presence of protein kinase activity in these granule preparations and that the proteins of these granules could be phosphorylated by protein kinase prepared from hypothalamus and pituitary. It also appeared that the neurosecretory granules could transfer phosphate to microtubular protein. Cyclic AMP were seen to stimulate these various phosphorylations. It was, therefore, postulated that when a secretory cell is stimulated, cyclic AMP-dependent changes in protein kinase activity could influence the interaction of neurosecretory granules and microtubules within the axon and nerve terminal, leading to release. Calcium ions could act to modulate these interactions. Against this suggestion, Thorn et al (1975) were unable to demonstrate any effect of dibutyryl cyclic AMP from the isolated rat neurohypophysis.

Parallel Release of Neurophysins and Neurohypophysial Hormones

The possibility that the release of neurophysin occurs simultaneously with that of the hormones, has stimulated a number of groups to develop radioimmunoassays for neurophysin. Tissot-Berthet, Reinharz and Vallotton (1975) developed assays for bovine neurophysin I and neurophysin II and used them to study circulating neurophysin in the human. They found in males a concentration of neurophysin I of 3.7 ± 1.5 (SD) ng/ml and of neurophysin II of 5.9 ± 1.9 ng/ml. They monitored neurophysin concentrations during the performance of a number of tests to stimulate the release of vasopressin, namely, the thirst test, the Cartter–Robins test (infusion of 700 ml 0.1M-Na C1) and the nicotine test. Only in the second test, where an osmolar load was given, was there a clear-cut response, a drop in neurophysin I and neurophysin II being seen.

Robinson (1975) developed assays for bovine neurophysins I and II and the two human neurophysins which he designated nicotine-stimulated neurophysin (NS neurophysin) and oestrogen-stimulated neurophysin (ES neurophysin). Normal plasma concentrations of NS neurophysin and ES neurophysin were found to be 0.9 ± 0.2 (SEM) ng/ml and 1.1 ± 0.004 ng/ml respectively. He found that the NS neurophysin was elevated in conditions when vasopressin secretion would be expected. There was, however, no clear relationship between oxytocin and ES neurophysin release. This last mentioned neurophysin is elevated throughout pregnancy but no change is seen during parturition. There is a mid-cycle peak during the menstrual cycle and elevated concentrations are seen in males with liver disease and renal disease. Despite this evidence Robinson did not feel justified in discarding the "one neurophysin - one hormone" hypothesis.

Legros (1975) has also developed specific radioimmunoassays for bovine neurophysin I and neurophysin II and has applied these assays to a series of investigations of neurohypophysial function. Although there are limits to the interpretation which can be placed on the results of such studies Legros feels that application of neurophysin radioimmunoassay will contribute much to the understanding of neurohypophysial function in the human. He obtained resting concentrations of neurophysin of around 2.5 ng/ml. These concentrations appear to fall with age, values of only 1.6 ng/ml being found in subjects of 50 - 60 years. He, too, reports an increase in immunoreactive neurophysin levels in pregnancy, although Tissot-Berthet et al (1975) were unable to demonstrate any change. Legros' observations on healthy subjects and on a number of patients led him to feel that simple determinations of plasma neurophysin are not a good index of neurohypophysial function. He felt rather that one should employ dynamic tests, as for example a water load test. Using this particular test on studies of inappropriate production of vasopressin, he was able to distinguish between patients in whom the hormone appeared to be produced by tumours and those with disturbances of central nervous system. Hamilton (1975) was able to establish the presence of neurophysin-like material in association with vasopressin activity in tumours from three patients with the syndrome of inappropriate vasopressin secretion. It seems that synthesis in tumours mimics that in the hypothalamus and that ectopic hormone production may arise from depression of normal genetic information present in cells. Additional studies of synthesis in tumours might well be of value in obtaining further information on the mechanism of vasopressin and neurophysin synthesis.

It has been suggested vasopressin may negatively feed back on its own release (see Chapter 8). Treatment of rats with pitressin tannate has also been shown to affect the neurophysin content of the posterior pituitary (Bakker, Dyball and Jones, 1975); thus, the pituitary neurophysin content increased after eight injections of vasopressin.

Information on the clearance of neurophysin and the neurohypophysial hormones has been provided by Johnston, Hutchinson, Morris and Dax (1975). They followed the disappearance of ^{125}I – labelled porcine neurophysin I and II from the plasma of the rat. They found a circulating half time in plasma ($t_{1/2}$) of neurophysin I was 1.5 min whilst that of neurophysin II was 1.7 min. Vasopressin and oxytocin were found to have a half time of similar length to these. Forsling, Martin, Sturdy and Burton (1973) also found a $t_{1/2}$ for vasopressin of 1.6 min but report that the $t_{1/2}$ for neurophysin to be 3.4 min. They, too, used radio-actively labelled neurophysin but the material was extracted from the bovine posterior pituitary.

Summary and Conclusions

In the years since neurophysin was first purified a great deal has been learnt about the nature of this group of compounds. They have frequently been used as markers for neurohypophysial hormones as they are easier to detect and measure. Thus, the hypothalamo-hypophysial pathways have been identified by labelling the neurophysin. It is not yet possible to replace hormone assays in plasma with assays of neurophysin, nor may it ever be. Much attention has been devoted to the mechanism of binding of the hormone to neurophysin. It appears that tyrosine 49 and a side chain carboxyl group of the neurophysin are important for binding.

Chapter 8

OSMOTIC CONTROL OF VASOPRESSIN SECRETION

"But, now that you've stated the whole of your case,
More debate would be simply absurd"

The primary controlling factor in the release of vasopressin is said to be the osmolality of the plasma. The system was defined by Verney (1947) who showed that in trained conscious dogs, infusion of hypertonic saline sufficient to produce a 1.8% change in plasma osmolality produced a reduction in water diuresis, which could be matched by an infusion of posterior lobe extract of 0.07mU/min. He postulated that the response was mediated through osmoreceptors which, by successive litigation of vessels, he located in the anterior hypothalamus. O'Connor (1962) has further shown a non-linear relationship between plasma osmotic pressure and release of vasopressin, hormone release being relatively greater with high osmotic pressures. Studies of Moses and Miller (1974) in which the plasma osmolality was altered by infusing 5% saline have indicated that in the human the osmotic threshold for release of vasopressin is 287 mOsm/Kg. Robertson (1974), using radioimmunoassay data, reports a threshold of 280 mOsm/Kg. Despite the fact that Verney published his findings nearly thirty years ago the exact site and nature of the receptors is still unknown. The more recent work of Anderson (1975) provides an alternative to the concept of osmoreceptors; he believes that the contribution of the blood brain barrier should not be neglected since it retards the penetration of most solutes to the CSF so that they dehydrate the brain, raising the concentration of sodium in the CSF. This in turn stimulates receptors in the vicinity of the third ventricle. Similar types of receptor are involved in ADH release and the response to thirst and it has been suggested that vasopressin itself may affect water intake. Much of this work has been concisely reviewed by Moses and Miller (1974) and Andersson (1975). Yoshida, Saito and Murase (1973) have also summarised this aspect of vasopressin release.

Possible Location and Nature of Osmoreceptors

Classically, nerve cells subserving various functions have been identified by ablation, stimulation, or recording of intracellular potentials. All three techniques have been used to identify the cells involved in the release of vasopressin. Hayward and his colleagues have performed a number of studies on the electrical activity of magnocellular neuroendocrine cells in the unanaesthetised monkey in various conditions. He has recently reviewed the results of these investigations (Hayward, 1974). Three types of cells identified by antidromic stimulation were classified on the basis of spontaneous firing pattern as "silent" (3%) continuously active (63%) and "burster" (21%). Hayward conjectured that the silent group represented cells in which synthesis and transport were the predominant activities. Those that were continuously active were cells in a state of tonic secretion while the final or burster group were those from which the hormone was released in a pulsatile fashion. Injections of hypertonic saline revealed a number of osmosensitive neurones which were divided into specific and non-specific cells. The specific osmosensitive cells were those cells located in the region of the supraoptic nuclei, which responded to an intracarotid infusion of sodium, but not to arousing sensory stimuli. The various cellular elements in the osmoreceptor-magnocellular complex were classified on the basis of their response to an osmotic stimulus as follows: specific biphasic (acceleration of discharge followed by inhibition) cells in the supraoptic nucleus which were considered to be the neuroendocrine cells, specific monophasic (acceleration or inhibition of discharge) cells in the perinuclear zone of the supraoptic nucleus which were considered to be the osmoreceptors of Verney and the nonspecific monophasic neurones which were considered to be the osmoreceptors of Sawyer and Gernandt (1956). It was suggested that this last set of receptors could be those involved in the behavioural aspects of osmotic stimulation such as drinking.

Earlier studies of Hayward revealed that areas outside the supraoptic nucleus, including the pre-optic area (Hayward and Barker 1968), could influence vasopressin release. Lesions in the septal and preoptic areas have been shown to affect fluid intake. Studies were therefore carried out by Van Gemert, Miller, Carey and Moses (1975) to see if these lesions in the hypothalamus acted directly on the thirst mechanisms or through ADH. Medial preoptic, lateral preoptic and septal lesioning was followed by a review of the fluid balance and vasopressin output in rats. Turnover of ADH was not affected by lesions in the lateral preoptic and septal regions, but was marginally increased in animals with medial lesions. The animals in this last group had a consistently elevated plasma osmolality, took in more fluid when water was freely available and their ability to conserve water during dehydration was reduced. This failure to conserve water appeared to result from unaltered vasopressin release during dehydration despite an increase in the plasma osmolality. This confirms the observations that there are several regions in the central nervous system, removed from the region of the supraoptic nucleus, which are capable of altering vasopressin release and hence water intake. The polyuria resulting from impaired vasopressin release during dehydration would result in a greater than usual increase in plasma osmolality and lead to polydipsia. An alternative explanation could be that the lesions altered the "setting" of the osmoreceptors, i.e. higher than usual plasma osmolality is required to stimulate vasopressin release.

Peck and Blass (1975) sought to identify the osmoreceptors involved in ADH release and the thirst response in rats by injecting a hypertonic solution of sucrose (0.60m Osm/Kg) in isotonic saline via chronically implanted cranial catheters. Urine flow in hydrated rats was used as the index of ADH release and the stimulus to drink was taken as the latency to drink after injection into the animal in a sleeping position. The results from 86 cannulae in 51 rats were presented; antidiuresis or drinking could be obtained from 44 of the placements scattered throughout the preoptic area of the anterior hypothalamus. The thirst and antidiuretic receptors were contiguous, but distinct; at only 15 placements were both antidiuresis and drinking elicited by intracranial injections. Generally the cannulae positive for drinking lay in the medial forebrain bundle and dorsal to the anterior hypothalamic area. Placements nearest the supraoptic nucleus did not elicit antidiuresis or give a strong drinking response. This data is compatible with the studies of Hayward in that osmoreceptors may be removed from the neurosecretory cells. It is impossible, however, to compare the studies as the two groups of workers sampled from different areas. The observations of Peck and Blass argue against Andersons 'blood brain barrier' hypothesis in that the former could induce ADH release and thirst stimulation by infusing a solution isotonic with respect to sodium ions but hyperosmotic by virtue of the added sucrose.

Intra-carotid Infusion of Solutions of Non-electrolytes

If the observations of Peck and Blass support the concepts of Verney then the studies of Olssen and Kolmodin (1974) appear to be incompatible with it. These workers studied the renal response of non-hydrated conscious goats to intra-carotid infusions of slightly hypertonic solutions (0.35M) of galactose, glycerol and fructose. Infusion was carried out fairly rapidly at a rate of 3.75 ml/min. The effect of all three agents was to produce a water diuresis which could be inhibited by ADH. The diuresis thus appeared to result from inhibition of ADH release. Volume changes did not seem to be involved as a similar volume of a saline solution did not alter free water clearance. Instead they postulate that the hypertonic infusions reduced the concentration of sodium in the CSF which in turn reduced the activity of the periventricular receptors and hence ADH secretion.

Osmoreceptors and Thirst

As already mentioned, osmoreceptors are also involved in the control of water intake. Since the thirst mechanism and vasopressin both act to maintain plasma volume it is not surprising that attempts have been made to find an interrelationship between the two systems. The possibility has been investigated by several workers including Szczepanska-Sadowska, Kozlowski and Sobocinska (1974). They describe experiments in which they observed the drinking response in intact and left side vagotomised animals. The threshold of drinking defined in terms of the drinking response to an osmotic stimulus (i.v. infusion of 0.75M NaC1) was reduced by subpressor amounts of vasopressin. This reduction was proportional to the dose infused over the range 22-47 μU/ml plasma. Vasopressin on its own never caused drinking. The concentrations of vasopressin reached in this investigation would not be found in normal circumstances, although they might occur in some patho-physiological conditions. The response was unaffected by left cervical sympathectomy. In contrast, infusions of pressor doses of vasopressin (406 μU/ml) elevated the drinking threshold to i.v. hypertonic saline infusion and this response was affected by cervical sympathectomy. It would seem that this second response results from vasoconstriction and displacement of the blood to central low-pressure areas. How AVP lowers the drinking threshold is not clear, but it could be due to increased excitability of the system controlling water intake in response to osmotic stimulation and/or modification of the permeability of the cell membrane of osmoreceptors.

Kozlowski and Szczepanska-Sadowska (1975) subsequently showed that volume expansion exerts an effect antagonistic to that of vasopressin on the thirst mechanism. The osmotic thirst threshold was increased by a 15% expansion of the blood volume produced by intravenous infusion of dextran solution. No significant change was seen when blood volume expansion was performed during infusion of vasopressin sufficient to produce a plasma vasopressin concentration of about 30 μU/ml in the expanded volume. It would thus look as though there is a complex relationship between plasma ADH, osmolality, blood volume and the thirst mechanism. These various parameters are integrated to maintain the body fluid volume within narrow limits.

Effect of Hypertonic Saline on Pituitary Neurohypophysial Hormone Content

Administration of vasopressin produces an effect not only on the thirst mechanism but also on the subsequent release of hormone from the pituitary (Bakker and Dyball, 1975). These authors first substituted a 2% sodium chloride solution for drinking water so causing a release of neurohypophysial hormones and consequent depletion of pituitary stores. Depletion was, however, reduced if the animals receiving 2% saline to drink were also treated daily with intravenous injections of 0.5% i.v. pitressin tannate. This could be explained if vasopressin exerted negative feedback on its own release. It could also be argued that treatment with vasopressin altered the baseline of these studies. However, the authors point out that animals treated with vasopressin did not drink less than 2% saline nor were the plasma osmolality or weight changes affected. That vasopressin can influence the hypothalamic-neurohypophysial system is confirmed by the observation that the neural lobe content of neurophysin is elevated in rats treated with exogenous vasopressin in Bakker, Dyball and Jones (1975). This effect could be brought about by influences on the synthesis or release.

Pituitary Vasopressin Content and Water Balance

The fall in pituitary content of vasopressin seen during the cellular dehydration, as induced by administration of 2% sodium chloride solution, raises the question of the quantity of vasopressin necessary for water balance. In contrast to many other hormones, considerable quantities of vasopressin are stored in the pituitary. Furthermore, it has been shown that water balance is maintained if only seven per cent of the neurohypophysial system is functioning. Young and Huang (1974) estimated the minimum quantity of pituitary vasopressin necessary for water balance in non-stressed rats. They used water intake as an index of vasopressin deficiency. The function of the neurohypophysial system was altered by electrolytic lesions in the hypothalamus and the resulting pituitary content was measured using both the pressor and antidiuretic assays. The lesions produced a precipitous drop in the vasopressin levels in the neural lobe over 3-5 days - 433 to 222 mU. The quantity of vasopressin necessary for water balance was found to be 50 mU or 8% of the normal pituitary content.

Summary

The location of the osmoreceptors involved in the release of vasopressin is not yet clear but it seems they do not necessarily lie in the region of the supraoptic nucleus. This system for AVP release has been shown to be closely related to the thirst mechanism and the hormone itself seems to exert a feedback on both systems. The data indicating osmoreceptor participation and those indicating sodium receptor involvement in the release of vasopressin are not yet reconciled.

Chapter 9

NON-OSMOTIC FACTORS IN VASOPRESSIN RELEASE

"And believes that they add to the beauty of scenes-
A sentiment open to doubt."

Vasopressin acts to promote water reabsorption and might therefore be expected to be released under conditions where conservation of water is desirable. Such situations might include reduction of circulating plasma or elevation of body temperature. Vasopressin release has been reported not only in these situations, but also under seemingly unrelated conditions of "stress". Considerable attention has been devoted to non-osmotic factors involved in vasopressin release and I suspect this is in part due to the nature of the assays which have not, on the whole, allowed detection of small changes associated with slight shifts in plasma osmotic pressure.

Haemorrhage is a potent stimulus of vasopressin release, producing some of the highest concentrations measured. Several groups of workers, including Share and Bisset and his colleagues, have investigated the underlying mechanisms. It is suggested that two types of receptor respond to hypovolaemia, although it is not known which one is dominant. These receptors are low pressure receptors located in the left atrium and high pressure receptors, namely the baroreceptors, in the carotid sinus and aortic arch. Much evidence for the involvement of intrathoracic volume receptors has come from the work of Henry and Gauer, who observed that distention of the left atrium was associated with a water diuresis. However, neither in their studies nor in those of several other workers, were estimates of plasma vasopressin made. The renal effects could therefore be due to other factors. Vasopressin release has also been reported in response to exercise, many types of stress and following anaesthesia and surgery. A factor common to these situations is the release of catecholamines and it has been suggested that they could act to release vasopressin. The results of Schrier (1974) however, suggest that the alterations in water excretion following adrenergic stimulation are mediated primarily by changes in baroreceptor tone and that vasopressin release is affected by afferent parasympathetic pathways.

The relationship of extracellular fluid to plasma vasopressin has recently been reviewed by Share (1974) who gives a commendably concise summary of the possible role of receptors in the cardiovascular system to vasopressin release and the relationship to catecholamines and cortisol. Schrier and Berl (1975), in summarising the non-osmolar factors affecting water renal excretion, also make mention of the influence of changes in blood volume and systemic arterial pressure. The role of atrial receptors in controlling the secretion of vasopressin and in the physiological regulation of body fluids has come under the scathing attack of Goetz, Bond and Bloxham (1975) who appear to find the evidence as satisfying as the evidence for a Loch Ness Monster! They have reviewed the subject and point out the limitations of the existing evidence. One major deficiency has been the satisfactory determination of vasopressin. In the absence of readily available assays workers have tended to rely on the response of the kidney in the experimental animal. This is not entirely satisfactory, for, as Forsling and Ullmann (1974b) have pointed out, there is no good correlation between vasopressin, urine flow and the ratio of urine to plasma osmolality. The development of more sensitive assays for vasopressin as described in Chapter 4 may help obviate this problem. Goetz et al also argue that many of the maneuvres designed to stimulate intrathoracic receptors, e.g. positive and negative pressure breathing, may not be as specific stimuli as hoped, since there may be associated changes in systemic haemodynamics. They commented on much other evidence and point out that in many of the experiments, where a relationship may have been proved, the changes in pressure induced may have been so great as to question the relevance to physiological situations.

Volume Receptors and Vasopressin Release

The controversy about the role of atrial receptors in the release of vasopressin continues. Much of the problem probably lies in the differences between the preparations used. Small changes in underlying conditions may well affect the responses including those in the kidney. Thus, while Kappagoda, Linden, Snow and Whitaker (1974) reported that relatively large doses of vasopressin are needed to produce antidiuresis in the anaesthetised dog, Forsling and Ullmann (1975a) found in situations where particular care is taken to ensure low vasopressin levels and the production of a true water diuresis, the canine kidney is responsive to very low concentrations of vasopressin.

In 1974 Kappagoda et al produced evidence to refute the role of atrial receptors in the release of vasopressin. They showed that the diuresis which accompanied left atrial distension did not appear to be accompanied by a fall in vasopressin in the plasma, but they did not perform a true assay on the plasma and the technique used was relatively insensitive. These workers however have gone on to show that the diuresis could still be obtained in the anaesthetised dog on stimulation of the atrial receptors, even after destruction of the posterior pituitary. The pituitary was ablated through a transsphenoid approach, using an electrocoagulator. They provide considerable histological evidence to show destruction of the pituitary and much of the adjacent hypothalamic tissue. The fact that they could not detect antidiuretic activity in the dog plasma is probably not significant in view of the assay used. The urine flow did not appear greatly different in those experiments in which the pituitary was ablated and the earlier experiments in which it was not. However, no measurements of GFR were made so that it is difficult to compare the studies. The left atrium in these studies was dilated by injecting warm saline into latex balloons inserted into the left atrium until the pressure had increased by about 15 mm Hg.

The diuresis associated with water immersion and which can be suppressed with vasopressin, has been taken as evidence of a role of atrial receptors. It is said that the expanded thoracic volume results in decreased vasopressin release. Epstein, Pins and Miller (1975) have confirmed that vasopressin secretion falls during water immersion of man. They followed the changes of urinary vasopressin, estimated by immunoassay and urinary excretory patterns, in well-hydrated volunteers before and during six hours immersion. Vasopressin excretion fell from a mean of 80.1 to 37.3 μU/ml (approx 200 pg/ml to 93.2 pg/ml) during water immersion. Excretion rapidly increased during the recovery hour when the subjects rested quietly outside the tank. These changes in AVP excretion were reflected by a significant rise during the recovery period. The plasma osmolality remained constant throughout the study. These results are therefore compatible with atrial receptor participation. It should be noted, though, as the authors themselves mention, that a number of haemodynamic changes occur including a fall in stroke volume and cardiac output with a drop in peripheral resistance. Vasopressin suppression could therefore be attributed to a change in baroreceptor activity.

Most workers have studied the effects of rapid changes in blood volume but Yesberg, Henderson and Budtz-Olson (1975) have studied the effect of a slow 12-15% reduction in blood volume over a period of days in sheep. This change occurred during a period of starvation, the study being performed to determine whether the fall in urine flow during starvation was a result of elevated vasopressin secretion. They could find no change in vasopressin concentration in the plasma nor any evidence for the involvement of aldosterone. It was therefore suggested that prolactin may be involved.

Shade and Share (1975) have reported further studies on blood volume and vasopressin release. They investigated non-hypotensive haemorrhage in anaesthetised dogs. There is some evidence that angiotensin may be involved in vasopressin release (Chapter 6). Shade and Share described a series of experiments carried out to ascertain whether increases in angiotensin II could potentiate vasopressin release in non-hypotensive haemorrhage. They found that angiotensin infusion had no effect on vasopressin at least during haemorrhage. This is in contrast to the osmotic stimulation of vasopressin which appears to be enhanced by angiotensin.

It is therefore suggested that volume and osmotic control of vasopressin are, to some degree, independent.

The possible effect of atrial receptors on water balance has been used to explain observations in various pathophysiological conditions such as congestive heart failure. A model system used to investigate sodium retention in this condition has been acute constriction of the thoracic inferior vena cava (TIVC), (e.g. Earley, Martino and Friedler, 1966). The mechanism of water retention was not investigated. Therefore Anderson, Cadnapaphornchai, Harbottle, McDonald and Schrier (1974) looked at the effect of TIVC constriction on renal water excretion. TIVC constriction was produced either using a snare around the TIVC or by inflation of a balloon placed in the cava via a femoral vein. The experiments were performed on four groups of dogs: - intact animals, acutely hypophysectomised animals receiving steroid replacement, hypophysectomized animals in which renal arterial and venous pressures were not controlled and animals in which the baroreceptors were denervated. In the intact dog TIVC constriction resulted in a fall in cardiac output and a diuresis. The renal arterial pressure and venous pressure were maintained by a clamp on the aorta and a snare on the abdominal vena cava and there was no alteration in the GFR. In the hypophysectomized dogs the drop in cardiac output was still observed but there was a reduced effect on free water clearance and urinary osmolality on constriction of the TIVC. In the hypophysectomized animals in which no compensation was made for changes in arterial and venous renal pressures there was no change in the urine osmolality although there was a drop in the free water clearance. In those animals with denervated baroreceptors there was no change in urine osmolality or free water clearance when the TIVC was constricted. These results were interpreted as showing that the changes in solute excretion are purely a result of changes in plasma vasopressin concentration, whereas the changes in urine excretion result from vasopressin release and reduction in distal fluid delivery. The authors, however, point out that this model is not completely analogous to congestive heart failure but corresponds to the hyponatraemic patient with cardiac failure.

Another observation which has been taken as evidence for atrial receptor participation is the increase in plasma vasopressin when subjects assume an upright position. Davies and Forsling (1975) have investigated this possibility by measuring vasopressin in the plasma of healthy volunteers who were tilted to 85° for up to 60 minutes, after resting supine for 90 minutes. Twelve subjects were used in the study and it was seen that in seven of the subjects there was little or no increase in vasopressin immediately after tilting but a small increase was noted about 45 minutes afterwards. The remaining five subjects experienced syncope or presyncopal symptoms and did not complete the study. On fainting, there was a pronounced increase in plasma vasopressin, a rise from 1.1 ± 0.1 (SEM) μU/ml to 11.0 ± 0.9 μU/ml. The changes in plasma vasopressin seen in the seven subjects completing the study did not coincide with the immediate changes in heart rate but did coincide with the period of maximum translocation of blood to the extremities. Sjostrand (1952) has shown that 600 ml blood of adult subjects is translocated to the legs around 20 minutes after assuming an upright posture.

Catecholamines and Renal Water Excretion

Schrier and his coworkers have produced a series of papers which indicate that there is an autonomic pathway involved in vasopressin release. Much of this evidence has been reviewed (Schrier, 1974; Schrier and Berl, 1975; Schrier, Berl, Harbottle and McDonald, 1975). Catecholamines are known to be able to produce a diuresis in some conditions and this could be brought about by suppressing the action of vasopressin on the kidney or by inhibiting its release. There is considerable evidence to show that catecholamines may act on cAMP in the kidney to alter renal excretion. Stimulation of β-adrenergic receptors increases cAMP concentrations causing an antidiuresis whereas α-adrenergic stimulation inhibits production of cAMP thereby reducing water reabsorption. Nevertheless Schrier and his colleagues have provided considerable evidence to show that an effect on vasopressin release must be considered. A dose of isoprenaline, found to produce antidiuresis if infused into the renal artery, failed to produce the same effect if given intravenously. Infusion of isoprenaline (0.04-0.06 μg/kg/min) into normal subjects produced a fall in blood pressure and an antidiuresis, and noradrenaline (600 μg/min) produced an increase in blood pressure and a diuresis without a change in GFR. No change was seen in the urinary excretion in subjects with diabetes insipidus (DI) infused with isoprenaline nor in DI subjects given a background infusion of vasopressin and noradrenaline (Berl, Harbottle and Schrier, 1974). It was therefore felt that α and β-adrenergic stimulation affect water excretion by exerting an effect on the release of endogenous vasopressin.

However, Forsling and Ullmann (1975b) made direct estimates of vasopressin in plasma following infusion of noradrenaline in the same dose that Schrier and Berl (1973) used. Plasma vasopressin fell in some animals and increased in others, but there was little overall change. Forsling and Ullmann however were unable to achieve stable cardiovascular parameters during the hour of infusion.

Schrier and his colleagues have also suggested that nicotine-induced release of vasopressin is produced by alterations in sympathetic tone rather than by a direct intracerebral effect. Thus Cadnapaphornchai, Boykin, Berl, McDonald and Schrier (1974) demonstrated that an intravenous injection of nicotine reversibly inhibited a water diuresis in dogs anaesthetised with pentobarbitone but not in acutely hypophysectomized dogs. No effect was seen either in animals in which the baroreceptors had been denervated. Direct intracarotid injections of nicotine were also ineffective in inhibiting water flow.

Schrier, Reid, Berl and Earley (1975) have also provided evidence that parasympathetic pathways are involved in renin release and have suggested that a fall in parasympathetic tone leads to an increased release of vasopressin which in turn suppresses renin secretion. This hypothesis is based on the observation that in intact anaesthetized dogs undergoing a water diuresis bilateral cervical vagotomy results in a fall in renin secretion and an increased urine osmolality, whereas in hypophysectomized dogs there was no change in plasma renin or urine osmolality.

Vasopressin Release after Anaesthesia and Surgery

Oliguria following anaesthesia and surgery is a well-known clinical problem. It has been suggested that this is a result of several factors, including an increased discharge of vasopressin. This latter has been ascribed, in part, to the action of anaesthetics which are said to stimulate vasopressin release. Forsling and Ullmann (1975a) have however, found that, with the exception of halothane, a number of anaesthetic agents did not prevent a water diuresis nor did they elevate plasma vasopressin. Inhibition of a water diuresis or vasopressin release were produced by operative trauma under inadequate anaesthesia, hypotension and arterial hypoxia.

Forsling and Ullmann (1974) went on to study the effect of arterial hypoxia on vasopressin secretion and on water diuresis in anaesthetised dogs. It was found that when the animals were artificially ventilated with 10% oxygen in nitrogen there was an increase in the circulating concentration of vasopressin of 32 ± 10.1 (SEM) μU/ml accompanied by prolonged oliguria and a rise in blood pressure. Pretreatment with guanethidine abolished the vasopressin response during hypoxia. It is well-known that stress results in an increased production of catecholamines, but the precise role of catecholamines in this response is not clear.

Forsling and Rees (1975) also report an increase in circulating vasopressin during hypoxia and hypercapnia in the anaesthetised cat. The animals were allowed to breathe spontaneously and after 5 minutes on 13% oxygen an average increase in plasma vasopressin of some 25.8 μU/ml was observed. Hypercapnia was also accompanied by a rise in plasma vasopressin provided the respiratory rate increased by more than 15%. No increase was seen if the respiratory rate did not increase significantly. It would seem therefore that vasopressin release under conditions of altered arterial gas tension in part depends on stimulation of thoracic receptors.

It is possible that this increased vasopressin release in conditions of lowered oxygen tension may be involved in high altitude pulmonary oedema. Therefore Singh, Malhotra, Khanna, Nanda, Purshottam, Upadhyay, Radhakrishnan and Brahmachari (1974) have investigated the changes in plasma vasopressin, catecholamines and cortisol in patients suffering from high altitude oedema. They found small increases in plasma vasopressin in patients just before and during the illness. More marked changes occurred in the cortisol concentration which showed a pronounced drop. The oliguria in these patients could thus be due to a drop in cortisol levels. The authors suggest that against the drop in cortisol, the small increase in plasma vasopressin could play an important role.

Temperature and Vasopressin Release

During exposure to high temperatures it would be of value to the animal to conserve water. There it might be expected that plasma vasopressin would be elevated in response to heating. Szczepanska-Sadowska (1974) showed that local heating of the hypothalamus led to increased vasopressin output. Forsling, Ingram and Stanier (1975) extended these observations using pigs to study the effect on vasopressin release of hypothalamic heating and cooling and of whole body heating. They used trained pigs with a thermode and thermistor implanted in the hypothalamus. When the pigs were placed in hot ambient conditions, such that there was a rise in rectal temperature, there was a rise in plasma vasopressin which could be abolished by cooling the thermode. Heating the thermode to 45°C had no effect on vasopressin concentration in neutral or cold temperatures, but produced a small rise at 35°C. There is thus clear evidence that vasopressin is released if an animal is exposed to high temperatures. This could arise from stimulation of thermoregulatory mechanisms or be secondary to other effects, such as the shift of blood to the peripheral circulation.

Sadowski, Kurkus and Chwalbinska-Moneta (1975) have investigated hormonal influences on renal function in dogs exposed to cold. These authors had previously reported an increase in plasma vasopressin in conscious dogs exposed to a cold environment. Despite the increase in plasma antidiuretic activity there was a fall in urine concentration, which they suggested could be due to an antagonistic effect of glucocorticoids on the kidney. They therefore studied changes in vasopressin, 17-hydroxycorticoids and noradrenaline in a group of dogs exposed to cold following treatment with metopirone, a potent inhibitor of cortisol biosynthesis. A problem in studying conscious dogs is that untrained dogs do not rest quietly during prolonged restraint, so in this second investigation the dogs were not restrained. It was found that the increase in vasopressin previously seen on exposure to cold was not observed in unrestrained dogs, but persisted in those dogs treated with an inhibitor of cortisol biosynthesis. It appears that in the conscious dog, cold can stimulate the vasopressin secretory mechanism, but that release is inhibited by plasma glucocorticoids. There is a complex series of hormonal changes in the cold, so that plasma AVP may decrease in man (Segar and Moore, 1968) or remain stable or increase as in the dog.

Summary and Conclusions

While changes in the plasma osmotic pressure are generally taken to be the chief stimuli for vasopressin release, other factors, particularly shifts in plasma volume and blood pressure, have been shown to play a role. However, considerable controversy surrounds atrial receptor involvement and a number of attacks on this hypothesis have been mounted during the year. As far as the blood pressure effect on vasopressin release is concerned, evidence has been assembled which suggests that parasympathetic activity may be involved in the control of vasopressin secretion. Many other factors have been implicated in the release of the hormone including temperature and hypoxia. The fact that changes in oxygen tension can affect circulating concentrations of vasopressin is of interest with respect to the physiological changes seen at high altitude.

Chapter 10

ACTION OF VASOPRESSIN ON AMPHIBIAN MEMBRANES

"Distinguishing those that have feathers, and bite,
From those that have whiskers, and scratch"

The mammalian kidney is a highly organised system with a multiplicity of functions. It is, therefore, very difficult to investigate the mode of action of a hormone at a cellular level in this organ. Model systems in which to study the mode of action have, therefore, been sought. Amphibian membranes have been deemed suitable models, especially the toad bladder. Vasopressin has two characteristic effects on this preparation, an increase in the permeability to water and an associated increase in sodium translocation. Vasopressin is believed to act first with membrane receptors, of which there are said to be two types; one associated with water transfer and the other with sodium. Vasopressin is only effective if applied to the serosal side, but the permeability barrier to water lies on the mucosal side so that a series of intracellular actions are implicated. Water transport is not believed to occur via the tight junctions. It is said to cross through the cells at the basal margin and by lateral intracellular channels. The exact nature of the permeable channels is not known but Ussing and his colleagues suggested that water passes through aqueous channels or pores, whose size is increased by neurohypophysial hormones. The stimulus-response coupling within the toad bladder is not fully understood but the ubiquitous adenosine 3', 5' monophosphate (cyclic AMP or cAMP) has been indicated to have a role. There is a considerable body of experimental evidence in support of this, including results from studies using cAMP, theophylline and direct measurement of cAMP. Thus on binding with the specific membrane receptor vasopressin activates adenylate cyclase and accelerates cAMP formation from adenosine triphosphate with the cell. Vasopressin sensitive adenylate cyclase has been prepared from toad bladders (Bar, Hechter, Schwartz and Walter, 1970), the only discordant observation being that this system is only stimulated by a concentration of hormone some hundred times greater than required to produce a response in the intact bladder.

For further details of these investigations the reader is referred to two reviews which have appeared recently; Hays and Levine (1974), although largely concerned with the mammalian nephron, summarise recent information on the toad bladder. A comprehensive review has appeared by Jard and Bockaert (1975) who, describing the stimulus-response coupling in neurohypophysial hormone target organs, concentrate on hormone/receptor interaction, subsequent stimulus generation and the relationship between stimulus generation and response.

Action of Vasopressin in Amphibia

The action of vasopressin on amphibian membranes is important in the overall water economy. It has been suggested that in general the intensity of the water balance response to neurohypophysial hormones is related to the terrestriality of the species. Hillman (1974) examined the effects of vasopressin on the urodele amphibian, *Aneides lugubris.* This salamander is highly specialised for terrestrial existence. Vasopressin brought about marked water retention in these creatures, resulting from the hydro-osmotic effects in the skin and bladder and the natriferic responses in the skin.

Action of Vasopressin on Cell Membranes

Although the toad bladder is commonly used as a model for vasopressin action, Park, Hong and Solomon (1975) recently introduced a note of caution. They found that treatment of toad bladder with amphotericin B inhibited the effect of vasopressin on osmotic water transfer. This substance had no such action on the kidney of rats with congenital diabetes insipidus. It should be said, however, that they used fairly high doses of vasopressin in the rat around 300 μU/min. However, it seems there are some circumstances where one cannot extrapolate from the toad bladder to the nephron.

Another point which has to be taken into account when considering the action of neurohypophysial hormones on amphibian membranes is that there appear to be independent pathways and hence separate underlying mechanisms for water and solutes. Reports appearing during the year have been consistent with this observation. Thus Pietras, Seeler and Szego (1975) found that pre-incubation of toad bladders with cortisol markedly reduces the increased water transport generally seen when vasopressin is added, but had no effect on the short circuit current, i.e. sodium transport response. Similarly Civan and DiBona (1974), studying electrical conductance across toad urinary bladder, demonstrated a separation of the natriferic and hydro-osmotic actions of vasopressin. Petrucelli and Eggena (1975) have confirmed the presence of independent pathways for urea and water transport. Tritiated water fluxes across the toad bladder in the presence of vasopressin were unaffected by the presence of cold thiourea, but the mucosal to serosal labelled urea fluxes were markedly retarded. Davis, Goodman, Schuster, Rasmussen and Martin (1974) investigated the effects of cytochalasin B on the response to vasopressin in the toad urinary bladder and found that this reagent produced marked increases in ^{14}C-urea movement without altering diffusional water permeability. The results of the same studies, however, are suggestive of a coupling mechanism between water and solute transport. As far as vasopressin stimulation of sodium transport is concerned, Huja, Szekerczes and Hong (1974) studying changes in short circuit current in isolated preparations of toad skin, suggest that the pathway for resting sodium transport is different from that followed after vasopressin stimulation.

It appears that the main barrier to water and solute transport is the luminal cell membrane and that vasopressin acts to alter its permeability. Interest has naturally centered on this membrane and the possible changes on addition of vasopressin. Wade, DiScala and Karnosvsky (1975) have applied the technique of freeze fracture electron microscopy to study the transporting epithelium of the toad bladder. This technique allows a view of the lipid interior of the membrane by producing fractures within the lipid portion of the membranes. The epithelium of toad bladder comprises four main types of cells (granule, mitochondria-rich, basal and goblet cells) of which the granular cells have been implicated in the response of the tissue to vasopressin and were of particular interest in this study. Striking differences between the luminal and basal membranes of these cells were reported including a difference in the size of intra-membranous particles, those on the luminal face being greater. Wade et al suggest, moreover, since these particles may represent islands of proteins within the lipid membrane they may become the system of pores already described for transfer of water and/or solutes. They have provided further evidence for this hypothesis from freeze fracture studies carried out on hormone treated cells. On exposure to vasopressin the membrane exhibited an ordered aggregation of the intra-membranous particles. The relative frequency of aggregation was closely correlated with the relative vasopressin-induced osmotic water flow suggesting that these ordered arrays of intra-membranous particles might represent the site of vasopressin stimulated water transfer. These structural changes of course could underlie changes in urea or sodium permeability. Civan and DiBona (1974) also carried out electron microscope studies to identify the site and mode of action of vasopressin. They noted changes in the profiles of cells (i.e. size) and differences in the intracellular space as an index to the movement of water and solutes. These studies were in parallel with observations on conductance changes induced by hypertonic solution bathing the mucosa, or hypotonic solution bathing the serosa, in the presence or absence of vasopressin. In this way the conductance of transepithelial pathways could be selectively altered. This powerful combination of tools was used to investigate the mode of hormone action. Changing the tonicity of the fluids bathing the membranes produces osmotic gradients which favours serosal to mucosal flux and hence conductance is raised. Production of these gradients also leads to increases of size within the limiting junctions and thus allows freer transepithelial ionic movement. Prior addition of vasopressin inhibits these effects causing a fall in osmotically induced conductance changes and a lessening of the blistering (i.e. spherical enlargement of intracellular spaces) seen at the apical junctions, shrinkage of the granular cells and vacuolation of all cell types in the mucosal epithelium. Thus vasopressin acts by increasing the permeability of the luminal facing plasma membrane, producing net movement of water across this membrane. It was also demonstrated that osmotic flow in response to vasopressin occurs through cells rather than between them, confirming there is no need to involve an effect of vasopressin at the junction when considering the action of the hormone. The results of these studies also strengthen the belief that granular cells are specifically involved in the hydro-osmotic effect, but do not throw light on the location of the natriferic effect.

Further evidence that the hydro-osmotic effect of vasopressin is largely exerted on the granular cells has come from the laboratories of Grosso, Spinelli and De Sousa. They have explored the problem by means of scanning electron microscope studies (Grosso, Spinelli and De Sousa, 1974; Spinelli, Grosso and De Sousa, 1974). They were able to identify, on the surface of bladders fixed with 2% gluteraldehyde three types of cell corresponding to the granular, mitochondria-rich and goblet cells. The granular cells were seen to have blunt microvilli, which diminished appreciably when vasopressin was applied in the presence of an osmotic gradient. No such change occurred in the microvilli of the smaller mitochondrial-rich cells. Identical results were obtained with cAMP and theophylline, both known to mimic the action of vasopressin. No change was seen if vasopressin was applied in the absence of a gradient so that it would seem water movement across the apical barrier is a pre-requisite for the disappearance of the blunt microvilli. Cytochalasin B, a macrolid antibiotic which selectively blocks the increase in hydro-osmotic permeability, but not sodium transport, produces a similar effect.

When toad bladder is treated with cAMP it has been shown that the granules in the cells at the luminal face, which may correspond to lysosomes, fuse with the apical membrane (Masur, Holtzman and Walter, 1972). Pietras, Seeler and Szego (1975) have taken these observations further and have shown that vasopressin produces a time dependent stimulation of release of lysosomal hydrolases from isolated epithelial cells, prepared from amphibian urinary bladder. This increment in the appearance of lysosomal enzymes was inhibited by the application of anti-vasopressin antiserum. Additional experiments performed on the intact bladder confirmed that release of lysosomal hydrolases occurred primarily from the mucosal surface.

Additional evidence that the action of vasopressin is associated with release of intracellular contents comes from the work of Taylor, Maffly, Wilson and Reaven (1975) who showed that cAMP stimulated the release of membrane limited granules at the apical surface of the granular cells. They suggest that the permeability changes are secondary to the release of granules by exocytosis and resultant inclusion of the granules into the existing membrane of the apical surface.

Another antimicrobial agent CM 55 which inhibits lipid synthesis has been used to look at sodium transport in the toad bladder: Ohno, Goodman, Rasmussen and Omura (1974) report that this agent inhibits vasopressin-stimulated sodium transfer. They therefore suggest that the response is dependent on continual turnover of lipid components. Glycoproteins, on the other hand, have been imputed to contribute to the urea transfer pathway. Sodium periodate, which probably acts by oxidizing surface carbohydrates, was shown to depress the permeability of the toad bladder to urea after the addition of vasopressin (Rubin 1975).

Displacement of bound calcium has also been implicated in the final processes responsible for permeability changes in the mucosa (Schwartz and Walter, 1968). Cuthbert and Wong (1974) developed methods for tracing the release of preloaded ^{45}Ca from preparations of isolated toad bladders. The technique allowed them to distinguish between release from serosal and mucosal surfaces. They were able to prove that calcium efflux does precede the natriferic and hydro-osmotic responses to vasopressin. Theophylline and prostaglandin E_1 also stimulated calcium efflux while lanthanum and amphotericin produced no change and cAMP inhibited calcium release. The increased release of ^{45}Ca was only from the mucosal surface and the calcium appeared to come from superficial sites in the mucosal membrane. The mechanism of release is not clear but the possibility of cAMP involvement cannot be ruled out. Sodium entry is not a pre-requisite for calcium release as the response is not altered by removal of sodium from the bathing medium or treatment with amiloride which blocks sodium transport.

Apparently there is no requirement for calcium in the vasopressin stimulation of sodium transport in the frog skin. Hall and Martin (1974) measured the short circuit current across frog skin after treatment with vasopressin or prostaglandin and found it was not affected by the addition of chelating agents or alterations in calcium concentration in the external bathing solution. Another conclusion derived from these studies was that prostaglandin and vasopressin act at the same site, as the maximal effect of one could not be augmented by the other.

Sodium transport across the toad skin appears to be coupled at least in part with excretion of hydrogen ions. Thus H^+ excretion increased after stimulation with antidiuretic hormone and decreased with amiloride (Emilio and Menano, 1975). Such an exchange could not be found across the frog skin, nor in the toad bladder (Frazier, 1974).

Cyclic AMP and Vasopressin Effects

So far the net effect of vasopressin on the membrane has been considered, but what of the intermediate stages? What occurs between binding of vasopressin to serosal membrane receptors and changes in the mucosal membrane? It is generally accepted that, in common with most other peptide hormones, vasopressin acts through cAMP. As already mentioned, the binding of the hormones to the receptors brings about activation of adenylate cyclase and generation of cAMP. This in turn stimulates protein kinases and it has been suggested that changes in phosphorylation of a membrane protein are involved in shifts of membrane permeability. Most observations can be explained on this basis. Mandel (1975), characterising the pathways for passive solute transfer across the skin, investigated the effect of urea and theophylline on the movement of extracellular solutes between and through apical cells. Vasopressin and theophylline in concentrations of 0.5 mM were found to increase transcellular movement of chloride whereas theophylline in a higher dose of 10 mM increased chloride transport both through and between cells. He explains these differences in terms of the concentrations of 3, 5 cyclic AMP generated in response to the agents.

Prostaglandin inhibits the effect of vasopressin on water flow in the toad bladder and it is believed that this modulating effect occurs through the adenylate cyclase step. One aspect of prostaglandin-vasopressin interaction which needs explanation is the finding that the inhibition by prostaglandin of the increased water flow, produced by vasopressin in quantities sufficient to bring about a maximal response, can be reversed by supramaximal doses of vasopressin. One possible explanation would be a reserve of vasopressin-sensitive adenylate cyclase as proposed by Eggena, Schwartz and Walter (1970). That is to say more adenylate cyclase is present that is necessary to produce a maximal increase in osmotic water flow. This suggestion is supported by data produced by Flores, Witkum, Beckman and Sharp (1974). They looked at the water flow, sodium transport and cAMP content of isolated toad bladder preparations. They report that a sharp increase in cAMP content was achieved with vasopressin, the maximum being seen at 8 min. The content of cAMP could be further elevated as greater concentrations of vasopressin were added (2.5×10^{-3}M to 20×10^{-2}M). At least three times more cAMP was generated by AVP than was required for full expression of its physiological action.

An unexpected observation made by Scott, Sapirstein and Yoder (1974) was that, although the granular cells appear to play a major role in transepithelial transfer, when epithelial cells were separated by density centrifugation, it was in the mitochondria-rich cell fraction that vasopressin induced increases in cAMP. Goodman, Bloom, Battenberg, Rasmussen and Davis (1975) applied the technique of immunofluorescent cytochemical staining to location of cAMP in toad bladder cells. Looking at sections of toad bladder tissue, they found that within two minutes of the application of vasopressin, cAMP content of both granular cells and mitochondria rich cells are increased.

It is suggested that cAMP may be transferred from mitochondria rich to granular cells as the tissue responds to vasopressin. Such interaction of cells in organ response to hormone is not unknown and in this case would account for the arrangement of cells described by Davis, Goodman, Martin, Matthews and Rasmussen (1974) - a rosette comprising one mitochondria rich cell surrounded by four or five granular cells.

Through studies on the action of many hormones on their target tissues, the characteristics of intracellular cAMP are well established. The relationship of changes in membrane permeability and phosphorylation of membrane protein is not so clear. Greengard and his associates, however, have provided us with some insight into the nature of the processes involved in sodium transfer. They indicated that both AVP and monobutyryl cAMP selectively decreased the amount of radioactive phosphate present in a phosphoprotein of apparent molecular weight 49,000 daltons, which they designated protein D. The time scale of dephosphorylation parallels that for changes in sodium transport. They pursued this promising lead by comparing changes in the phosphate content of this protein with changes in sodium transport (Walton, De Lorenzo, Curran and Greengard, 1975). The membrane proteins were separated using SDS polyacrylamide electrophoresis and followed by estimating the amount of radioactive protein using autoradiography and microdensitometry. To stimulate transfer of sodium, the following were employed: ADH, cAMP, theophylline, adenine, prostaglandin E and magnesium chloride. These agents produced an effective dephosphorylation (i.e. a decrease in the amount of ^{32}P phosphate present in the 49,000 dalton protein). Zinc chloride which produces an inhibition in sodium transport had the reverse effect. Further the change in phosphorylation followed the same time scale as the change in sodium transport and was correlated with the natriferic potency of the particular agent. There was no relationship with alterations in osmotic water permeability. Similar changes were also found in the radioactive phosphate content of a second protein of molecular weight 42,000 dalton.

On the basis of these observations, Walton et al propose a model for the regulation of sodium transport by ADH and cAMP. They feel that sodium transport is in no way related to changes in protein phosphate as amphotericin treatment reduced short circuit current to a fraction of control but had no effect on phosphorylation of these specific proteins. Instead they hypothesize that cAMP acts on the permeability of the membrane to sodium. The membrane could exist in two states, one in which it is highly permeable to sodium and another in which it is relatively impermeable. The region of high permeability would be that in which the protein existed in the dephosphorylated state, cAMP would thus act by stimulating a protein phosphatase which acts on the 49,000 dalton protein and perhaps on the 42,000 dalton protein. The net effect of ADH would be a shift in favour of the dephosphorylated protein and hence a change in sodium transport.

Interrelationship between vasopressin and water balance in amphibia now appears more complicated than originally thought. Eggena, Christakis and Deppisch (1975) have shown that overhydration reduces the responsiveness of the urinary bladder to AVP suggesting that body fluid balance depends not only on osmotic control of the release of vasopressin, but also on the osmotic regulation of the action of the hormone.They believe this to be a result of reducing the effective concentration of cAMP following AVP stimulation. Phase contrast microscopy revealed that isolated cells of the epithelium behaved as perfect osmometers, doubling their volume as the osmolality of the medium halved. Thus although AVP stimulated cAMP production, so that the cell content increases three to five times, the content in the cells in hypotonic solution was effectively diminished. Thus cAMP may be involved in the altered responsiveness of cells to vasopressin in conditions which engender osmotic swelling.

Aldosterone

The effective concentration of cAMP is altered by many factors other than dilutional effects. Alterations in the activity of the enzyme phosphodiesterase which destroys cAMP produce this effect. Adrenal steroids are said to act this way. Orloff, Handler and Stoff (1973) have shown that preincubation of toad hemi-bladders with aldosterone enhanced osmotic flow and the sodium transport response to treatment with cAMP or vasopressin. The fact that similar effects were produced by both cAMP and vasopressin suggested that the response to the latter involves the nucleotide. Evidence that the phenomena entailed the pathways of degradation of cAMP was given by its enhanced accumulation in aldosterone treated bladders in response to vasopressin. Hewitt, Debnam and Snart (1975) believe that there are two sets of mineralocorticoid receptors on the toad bladder, one of which is involved in phosphodiesterase inactivation. They found that the response to low doses of vasopressin could be enhanced by 10^{-7}M aldosterone.

Cuthbert and Shum (1975) have also studied changes in the permeability characteristics of toad bladder on treatment with aldosterone and vasopressin. They have not studied the potentiation of vasopressin performance, but their observations throw light on possible mechanisms. Their results appear to show that aldosterone and vasopressin stimulate sodium transport by separate pathways as Sharp and Leaf (1966) also concluded. Cuthbert and Shum used the binding of (^{14}C) amiloride as a marker of sodium transport sites. This substance has been shown to block entry in a number of membranes and is therefore a useful molecule with which to probe sodium transport phenomena. Using this compound they deduced that aldosterone acts by producing more available sites for sodium transport. Vasopressin on the other hand does not affect the number of sites available for translocation but would appear to act by increasing the number of available sites actually involved in transport. This scheme could explain the mineralocorticoid potentiation of vasopressin without the necessity of invoking changes in cAMP turnover.

Cyclic AMP has also been imputed to play a part in the action of the diuretic agent ethacrynic acid (Ferguson and Twite, 1975). This is in contrast to several other agents. Thus ethacrynic acid produces a fall in cAMP levels and depresses the increase on vasopressin stimulation. Axman and Fulgraff (1975) have looked at the action of another diuretic, furosemide, on frog skin. They found that it shares a common action with vasopressin in that it stimulates sodium entry into the transport compartment of the cell layer.

Role of Microtubules in the Vasopressin Response

While changes in membrane protein phosphorylation are said to transduce cAMP stimulated changes in sodium permeability, microtubules appear to be involved in alterations of water flow. As already described, secretory granules from granular cells discharge their contents upon vasopressin stimulation. It is possible that this is brought about through the mediation of microtubules. This intracellular system of microtubules and microfilaments has excited the interest of endocrinologists and this general interest has been extended to vasopressin. A means of investigating the involvement of microtubules is through the use of agents such as colchicine and cytochalasin B. The structural effects of the latter compound have already been discussed. It has been shown in many systems to cause disorganisation of the cytoplasmic cell web, thereby influencing several cell functions. De Sousa, Grosso and Rufener (1974) have confirmed that cytochalasin B blocks the osmotic effect of vasopressin, but does not affect sodium transport. They put forward two explanations - cytochalasin B could either affect the permeability to water of the apical membrane or could disrupt microfilaments, thereby affecting secretion of stimulus coupling of the neurohypophysial hormones.

Taylor and Reaven (1975) have demonstrated that colchicine inhibits the action of vasopressin transcellular water movement in toad bladder. They proceeded to study ultrastructural changes produced by this agent using electron microscope studies. The effect of vasopressin was also investigated. The density of microtubules in cells from toad bladder was decreased by colchicine (2 x 10^{-6}M to 8 x 10^{-4}M) whereas it was increased by vasopressin (100 mU/ml). Thus vasopressin influences the organisation of microtubules in granular cells and colchicine inhibits the vasopressin response through interference with the assembly of microtubules. This is in keeping with the second suggestion of De Sousa et al (1974).

Summary

Vasopressin acts on certain amphibian membranes to cause profound changes in the structure of the epithelial cell layer and an increase in the transfer of solute and water. This is achieved through the mediation of cAMP and the properties of this system have been further elucidated. Alterations of sodium translocation may be brought about by changes in membrane permeability secondary to dephosphorylation of certain membrane proteins. Hydro-osmotic changes may reflect underlying effects on the microtubules; this may entail exocytosis from the granular cells and subsequent incorporation of the membrane into the apical surface membrane. It is also interesting to speculate that vasopressin, by causing contraction of the microtubules, may have a similar effect in the fluid maintenance and cardiovascular responses.

Chapter 11

RENAL ACTIONS OF VASOPRESSIN

"Fell asleep, and in dreams saw the creature
quite plain
That his fancy had dwelt on so long."

Surprisingly the first reported action of vasopressin on the kidney was diuresis (Magnus and Schafer, 1901). It is now well established that the hormone can produce this effect, but at concentrations normally found in plasma it acts chiefly on the distal convoluted tubule and collecting duct to increase permeability and allow water to move down the concentration gradient in the kidney. Vasopressin acts on the cells of renal tubule from the basal (blood) side but alters the permeability on the apical (urinary) side. Grantham and Burg (1966) have suggested that the response is brought about by an increase in the number of pores allowing passage of water. As described in Chapter 10, current concepts of the mechanism of vasopressin action have come from the study of amphibian membranes. Vasopressin first acts with receptors near the peritubular surface which have a very high specificity for vasopressin. Thus vasopressin is effective in very low concentrations. For example, in the rat a dose of 100 μU/100 g produces a marked antidiuresis. As with the toad bladder, it is suggested that binding of the hormone to the membrane is associated with activation of adenyl cyclase which in turn results in an elevation of intracellular cyclic AMP (cAMP). This initiates a further series of reactions which results in an increase in cell permeability. Much of this evidence is summarised by Sawyer (1974) and Kurtzman and Boonjaren (1975). The renal response to vasopressin is further affected by electrolyte balance and by a number of hormones including adrenaline and the prostaglandins. Some of these interactions are summarised by Naftalin (1975).

Site of Action

In 1952, Smith suggested that re-absorption of water without solute occurred in the distal part of the nephron. Subsequent micropuncture studies by Wirz (1957) and others lead to the conclusion that vasopressin acts to increase the permeability to water of the distal tubule and possibly also the collecting duct. It appears that in the rodent vasopressin acts on the distal tubule (e.g. Wirz 1957) whereas in the dog and the rhesus monkey it appears to act more distally - in the collecting duct. Studies on isolated perfused sections of the nephron have allowed the site and nature of the response to be more clearly defined. Abramow and Dratwa (1974b) have perfused the isolated collecting duct of rabbit with hypertonic buffer using ^{125}I-iothalamate, a volume marker to measure net transfer. They were able to demonstrate a marked increase in this parameter in the presence of vasopressin. These workers later studied the effect of vasopressin in the isolated human collecting duct, taken from a 5.5 month male foetus (Abramow and Dratwa, 1974c). In this preparation also, they were able to demonstrate a marked increase in osmotic water permeability after the addition of vasopressin (2.13 mU/ml) to the bathing medium. This increased water permeability was accompanied by morphological changes, including swelling of the cells, vacuolation and dilation of the intercellular spaces. This would suggest that water movement here also occurs through intercellular channels in addition to the cell membrane.

Rocha and Kokko (1974) have studied the effect of vasopressin on the permeability of the medullary nephron segments to urea and water. This was part of a more extensive study on urea circulation within the medulla. Kokko had already shown that in the rabbit the thin descending limb of the loop of Henle is impermeable to urea, but permeable to water and that the thin ascending loop was slightly permeable to urea and impermeable to water. Therefore in these next experiments they studied the characteristics of the thin ascending loop of Henle and the outer medullary collecting duct. They were able to confirm that the medullary thick ascending limb of the loop of Henle was impermeable to water even in the presence of vasopressin. The permeability of the papillary collecting duct increased if 200μU/ml vasopressin were added to the bathing fluid. This section of the collecting duct also showed some permeability to ^{14}C urea but this was unaffected by vasopressin.

Changes in the Sensitivity of the Kidney to Vasopressin

A number of factors have been said to reduce the renal sensitivity to vasopressin. Kingsley, Goldberg, Abrahams, Meyers, Furman and Cohen (1972) have described changes in the urinary concentrating ability of the kidneys after prolonged administration of analgesics containing phenacetin. Ratnikow (1975) has performed a series of observations on this phenomenon in the dog. Animals were treated for six months with either acetyl salicylic acid (100 mg/kg), sodium salicylate (200 mg/kg) or phenacetin (80 mg/kg). At the end of this period pituitrin injections were less effective in inhibiting antidiuresis in all these groups of animals than in control animals. The studies however revealed little of the underlying changes.

The observations that sheep with vitamin A deficiency excrete increased volumes of a relatively more dilute urine compared with normal animals has been examined by Ritter, Tucker, Schelling and Mitchell (1975). They believe that lack of vitamin A causes renal damage which affects the renal concentrating mechanism by reducing the renal sensitivity to vasopressin.

Role of Cyclic AMP

There is considerable experimental evidence to suggest that cAMP acts as a mediator of vasopressin induced changes in the water permeability of amphibian membranes (Chapter 10). A similar mechanism is proposed for the mammalian nephron. The entire sequence of events is triggered by the binding of vasopressin to the receptor. Imbert, Chabardes and Morel (1975) and Imbert, Chabardes, Montegut, Clique, Morel and Courrier (1975) have used measurements of adenyl cyclase to confirm the site of vasopressin receptors in the nephron. They used recently developed micromethods to determine adenyl cyclase in 1 mm lengths of rabbit nephron. They found that vasopressin stimulated adenyl cyclase activity in the collecting duct but had no effect on the distal convoluted tubule and thin descending loop. This is surprising since the distal convoluted tubule has been postulated to be the site of vasopressin action. These results therefore cast doubt on this hypothesis but do not exclude the possibility that the very last part of the distal convoluted tubule is sensitive to vasopressin. However, they observed a marked effect in the outer medullary thick ascending limb, but at higher vasopressin concentrations than were effective on the collecting duct. The significance of these findings remains to be established, but they do raise the question of two different sites of action of vasopressin in the nephron. The additional effect might well be on sodium transport.

Imbert, Chabardes, Montegut, Clique and Morel (1975) extended these studies and looked at the various sections of the collecting duct; the branched cortical part, the cortical straight part and the outer medullary part. They were able to demonstrate a highly sensitive adenyl cyclase in all parts of the collecting duct. The range over which the dose response curve for the adenyl cyclase response extended was much greater than for the antidiuretic response. Thus the lowest concentration which produced an increase in cAMP production was 10^{-11}M (or approximately 5μU/ml) which is of the order required to produce a biological response in the intact animal. However the maximum response was obtained at 10^{-7}M. It is not obvious why the adenyl cyclase in the collecting duct should respond to vasopressin concentrations well outside those occurring normally.

Jard and his colleagues have done much to characterise the vasopressin receptor: Jard, Roy, Rajerison, Barth and Bockaert (1974) and Roy (1974) have prepared membrane fractions from pig renal medulla. This preparation was shown to possess adenyl cyclase activity which could be stimulated by lysine vasopressin (LVP); the response was accompanied by binding of LVP, activation of adenyl cyclase and uptake of tritiated LVP following the same time course. The relationship was not however linear. Further the response depended on the particular analogue used. Thus oxytocin was not as effective in stimulating adenyl cyclase. Jard, Roy, Barth,

Rajerison and Bockaert (1975) presented two hypotheses to account for the non-linear coupling. The first is a "multistep activation process" in which the activation of adenyl cyclase is a saturatable function of an intermediate formed on hormone–receptor interaction. In the second, adenyl cyclase is activated as a result of some propagated structural changes within the membrane, produced as a result of hormone receptor interaction. Roy, Rajerison, Bockaert and Jard (1975) have further examined the properties of inactivation with Triton x-100. Although the yield for adenyl cyclase was 100%, that for the receptors was only 30% and the apparent affinity of LVP for the solubilized receptor was five times lower than the affinity for the receptor when it was within the membrane.

Additional characterisation of the receptors has been attempted using vasopressin analogues (see also Chapter 3). Cort, Skopkova, Schuck, Stribrna and Sawyer (1975) have used three types of vasopressin analogues in human volunteers and in rats. These were analogues with aliphatisation in the ring; those with substitution of a CH_2 group in the disulphide bridge (carba-derivatives) and those with alterations in position 8 of the C-terminal tripeptide. As a result of their studies Cort et al suggest that there is a specific antidiuretic receptor in the kidney. The disulphide bond appears to play a part in the receptor hormone interaction. Aliphatisation altered the affinity for the receptor as did steric changes in the terminal tripeptide.

Extensive studies on the reaction of analogues with pig kidney preparations have been carried out by Roy and Jard and their colleagues. As indicated above, they believe that there is non-linear coupling between the receptor occupancy and the adenyl cyclase response. Similar patterns of response however could be obtained if there were a heterogeneous population of receptors, only some of which have a high affinity for LVP. In order to clarify the situation, Roy, Barth and Jard (1975) and Jard et al (1975) looked at the response of vasopressin sensitive adenyl cyclase to a number of different analogues. They found a good correlation between activation of adenyl cyclase by the various analogues and the ability to displace bound, tritiated LVP. This indicates that the binding sites revealed in these studies are probably the physiological receptors involved in adenyl cyclase activation. It furthermore indicates that these isolated membrane fractions retain a high degree of specificity with respect to vasopressin receptors. More specifically, these studies revealed great differences in the peptides studied, these being a variation in the magnitude of maximal stimulation, apparent affinity (i.e. the concentration of hormone giving half maximum saturation) and the shape of the dose response curve. Just as Cort et al (1975) showed *in vivo* so these workers were able to show that two carba-derivatives deamino-6-carba- (D Arg^8) vasopressin and (Tyr $(Bu^t)^2$ Arg (Tos^8) deamino-6-carba vasopressin produced a greater stimulation than LVP itself. The apparent affinity varied over a wide range from 2.5×10^{-10}M for LVP to over 10^{-4}M for pressinamide. These observations paralleled the structure activity relationships reported in Chapter 3, namely, that a disulphide bond is not necessary for the binding of the hormone to the receptors, that substitution of an amide group in position 1 enhances the apparent affinity for the receptor and that there is a correlation between affinity and basicity of the side chain. The fact that there was identical maximum displacement of LVP by the active analogues and that the time course of binding and reversibility are adequately described in terms of binding of hormone to a homogeneous population of binding sites indicates that there is a uniform population of receptor sites.

Since preparations of renal adenyl cyclase appear to be so useful in determining the factors governing interaction of hormone with renal receptors, the studies were extended to analogues with enhanced or prolonged activity *in vivo* (Barth, Roy, Rajerison and Jard, 1975; Barth, Rajerison, Roy and Jard, 1975). They first tested the activity of amino acylated vasopressin and oxytocin. Addition of an amino acid or a short peptide residue to produce, for example, (N[glycyl-Cys-] 8-lysine) vasopressin reduces the biological activity. Nevertheless these analogues commonly can produce a protracted response. It is believed that the parent molecule is gradually released from these less active analogues *in vivo* (Kyncl and Rudinger, 1972). The LVP and oxytocin analogues tested were able to activate renal adenyl cyclase preparations from pig or rat tissue, but they exhibited lower maximum activity than the parent molecule. There was good correlation between activity in this system and that *in vivo*. It appeared that the activation of adenyl cyclase was produced by the substituted peptide itself, since, on incubation with kidney medullary membranes from the rat, the parent molecule did not appear to be released.

Amongst the modifications which enhance antidiuretic activity are deamination of cysteine in position 1 and substitution of D-for L-arginine. Such a derivative is deamino D-Arg^{8}-vasopressin (see Chapter 3). Barth et al (1975) have looked at the activity of a number of such analogues and carba-derivatives. These analogues were not more potent than the naturally occurring hormones in activating renal adenyl cyclase nor were they degraded during incubation with renal membranes. This confirms that the increased *in vivo* activity results from enhanced metabolic stability.

Barnes, Hui and Dousa (1975) have demonstrated an interaction of ethacrynic acid and cysteine with renal medulla adenyl cyclase. They were able to demonstrate that ethacrynic acid and its cysteine adduct were able to inhibit basal and vasopressin stimulated adenyl cyclase. The sulphydryl grouping was not a pre-requisite for inhibition, but it was thought that it could contribute in some way. Cysteine, on the other hand, potentiated adenyl cyclase activity. It was suggested that ethacrynic acid acts on the collecting ducts to block vasopressin action by inhibiting the catalytic sub unit of cyclase (Hui, Barnes and Dousa, 1975).

In addition to studies on vasopressin receptors and the character of adenyl cyclase, observations have been made on the steps subsequent to activation of adenyl cyclase, including possible phosphorylation of membrane proteins. Barnes, Hui, Frohnert and Dousa (1975) have studied enzymes associated with the cellular action of vasopressin. They studied the subcellular distribution in preparations of bovine renal medulla of four enzymes - adenyl cyclase, cAMP phosphodiesterase, protein kinase and protein phosphorylase. This information is needed for fuller understanding of the reactions involved in producing the vasopressin response. Vasopressin stimulated adenyl cyclase was found almost exclusively in plasma membranes. The dose of vasopressin required to produce stimulation was of the same order as seen in preparations from other species. The other enzymes investigated were localised in the cytosol. In this preparation cAMP in quantities of 10^{-6} to 10^{-4}M had no effect on the protein phosphorylase. This is in contrast to the toad bladder, where cAMP dependent protein dephosphorylation appears to be involved in vasopressin stimulated sodium transport. It could be that these reactions are solely involved in sodium transport and are not required in the kidney for the vasopressin mediated changes in permeability. Regarding the overall system it is likely that these various soluble enzymes are held in a specific location or transferred to their membrane substances by a series of microtubules.

Rayson and Morgan (1975) have confirmed that the increase in water permeability produced by vasopressin depends on the adenyl cyclase -cAMP system, but suggest that there are other sites involved in the response. Thus in the presence of 7.2mM Mg^{++} vasopressin produced a greater stimulation of adenyl cyclase activity than at 1.2 mM Mg^{++}, but a reduced increase in the cAMP content and diffusional water permeability of the collecting duct of the rat kidney.

Modification of the antidiuretic action of vasopressin in a number of situations has now been explained through an effect on cAMP in the kidney. It has been reported that acidic media inhibit the hydro-osmotic effect of vasopressin on the toad bladder (Rasmussen, Schwartz, Young and Aurele, 1963). The evidence for the involvement of cAMP is open to question. Beck and Kim (1975) have therefore investigated the inhibiting mechanism in rat kidneys. They were able to assert that tubular re-absorption of free water in response to vasopressin was inhibited by acute metabolic acidosis and that less cAMP was excreted in the urine. Similarly, in a series of *in vitro* experiments in which the responses of renal medullary slices were observed, it was noted that the increase in cAMP concentration and the activation of adenyl cyclase induced by vasopressin was considerably less when the tissue was bathed in an acidic medium. However, acidic media could inhibit cAMP phosphodiesterase, so that as well as inhibiting the vasopressin-dependent cAMP system, acidosis could also increase cAMP concentration by inhibiting its breakdown. This could explain the controversial findings using the toad bladder.

Potassium depletion is also known to inhibit vasopressin response in the rat kidney. It has been shown, both by *in vivo* and *in vitro* techniques that this is, at least in part, due to an effect on cAMP (Reed and Beck, 1975; Beck, Reed and Davis 1975). The impaired urinary concentration occurring during hypercalcaemia has also been ascribed to an effect of calcium on adenyl cyclase. Beck, Singh, Reed, Murdaugh and Davis (1974) found that hypercalcaemic rats exhibited a reduced antidiuretic response and a reduction in cAMP excretion after vasopressin injection as compared with a control group. Activation of adenyl cyclase by vasopressin *in vitro* was also reduced in tissue from hypercalcaemic animals.

Microtubules and the Vasopressin Response

An exciting observation linking changes in cAMP concentration with other cellular events possibly induced in the response to vasopressin has come from Barnes and Dousa (1975). They were able to show that tubulin prepared from both bovine renal medulla and pig brain could polymerize *in vitro* to produce microtubules. This event could be inhibited by 0.1 mM cAMP. As with response of the toad bladder to vasopressin so in the mammalian kidney it is conjectured that microtubules play a role. The procedure for the *in vitro* polymerisation of tubulin from the bovine renal medulla is described in detail by Barnes, Engel and Dousa (1975). In essence, formation of microtubules from tubulin is achieved in renal medullary cytosol, following concentration by ultrafiltration, and incubation in the presence of ethylene glycol bis(2-aminoethyl)ether tetra-acetic acid and 4M glycerol. The presence of tubules was elegantly illustrated by electron microscopy. Microtubule assembly was blocked by vinblastine (10^{-10}M) and by a small increase in ionized calcium. This accords with *in vitro* observations that elevated extracellular calcium concentrations block the hydro-osmotic response to vasopressin (Argy, Handler and Orloff, 1967).

Abramow and Dratwa (1974a) have briefly reported on their data on the effects of cytochalasin B (which acts on microtubules) on the isolated collecting tubule of the rabbit. As a result of their studies they believe that the bulk transfer of water following vasopressin may be facilitated by changes in the microtubules. Further support for this hypothesis has come from Hall, Taylor and Maffly (1974) who pursued the inhibition of vasopressin action by colchicine, an agent which disrupts cytoplasmic microtubules. They used rats with hereditary diabetes insipidus. Colchicine had no effect on the production of dilute urine in these animals, but did impair the response to vasopressin.

Prostaglandins and Vasopressin Action

Prostaglandins have been implicated in the regulation of hormonal action in a number of tissues including the toad bladder where prostaglandin E_1 (PGE_1) has been shown to oppose the hydro-osmotic action of vasopressin. Similar effects have been shown in the rabbit collecting duct (Grantham and Orloff, 1968). Anderson, Berl, McDonald and Schrier (1975) have attempted to demonstrate the phenomenon *in vivo*. Instead of infusing prostaglandin which would have produced a number of unwanted effects, they studied the actions of inhibitors of prostaglandin synthesis on the response to vasopressin in acutely hypophysectomized dogs who had received steroid replacement and were undergoing a water diuresis. Two inhibitors with different types of action were used, indomethacin and meclofenamate. It was found that in the presence of either inhibitor the antidiuretic response to vasopressin was considerably enhanced. Thus an injection of 100 mU vasopressin raised the urinary osmolality from 92 to 252 mosmol/kg water, but in the presence of indomethacin the increase was from 106 to 702 mosmol/kg water. These studies however did not indicate the site of action so that vascular or cellular responses could be involved.

Berl, Horowitz, Czaczkes, Wald and Kleeman (1975) made a similar series of observations in both human volunteers and in rats. Thus in man, in the presence of indomethacin the antidiuretic response to vasopressin was much more marked. This effect was independent of changes in solute, inulin or PAH clearances and was not correlated with changes in cAMP secretion. A similar effect was seen in rats given subcutaneous injections of 250 mU vasopressin in oil and 10 mg/kg/day indomethacin on two consecutive days. Creatinine excretion was unchanged in these animals and analyses of preparations of renal cortex, medulla and papilla revealed no changes either in phosphodiesterase or adenyl cyclase activity. In contrast to the many other responses already discussed, it appears that in this case cAMP does not play a role.

Effects of Vasopressin on Solute Excretion

Schafer first described the diuretic action of vasopressin and ascribed it to a possible vascular effect. Since that time a modest number of reports have appeared on the diuretic animals. Some of this information has been summarised by Lee and de Wardener (1974). Kurtzman, Rogers, Boonjaren and Arruda (1975) have investigated this problem in dogs, giving vasopressin infusions of 50 mU/kg/min or 50 mU/kg/h. Three groups of animals were studied: bicarbonate-loaded, glucose-loaded and non-loaded dogs in a state of antidiuresis. Despite the difference in the amounts administered, both dose levels produced an increase in sodium, chloride and urea excretion.

Attempts to locate the cause and site of action showed that it was not a result of the hypertensive effect of vasopressin, as the changes in solute excretion were still seen when the pressor effects were blocked with sodium prusside. Changes in glomerular filtration rate and renal blood flow could not therefore be involved. Renal haemodynamic changes were ruled out following measurements of cortical renal blood flow with microspheres. Kurtzman et al believed that vasopressin was acting proximally in this preparation as glucose, bicarbonate and phosphate reabsorption were unaffected. They concluded that the most likely cause of the diuresis was an effect on electrolyte transport in the nephron, at a site distal to the proximal tubule.

Hiatt, Miller and Katayanagi (1975) were able to demonstrate a diuretic effect of vasopressin on dogs infused with 2 mmol/kg/min KCl. As might be expected these animals developed pre-lethal cardiotoxicity in about 3 hours, but vasopressin delayed the onset to about 5 hours. It was suggested therefore that vasopressin in this case was playing a role in potassium homoeostasis. Conversely, in rats with hereditary diabetes insipidus which have been shown to have potassium deficiency, subcutaneous injections of around 100 mU of vasopressin in oil produced potassium retention (Mohring, Mohring, Schomig, Schomig-Brekner and Haack, 1974).

In addition to an effect on sodium excretion, Slepushkin (1975) showed that in dogs undergoing a water diuresis, vasopressin over a wide range of doses (0.5 - 80 mU/kg) produced increased excretion of magnesium and calcium. Vasopressin has also been shown to affect sodium excretion through interaction with the renin angiotensin system (Al-Merani, Chapman and Munday 1974). Thus the reduction of sodium excretion, induced by infusing 20 mg/min angiotensin, was inhibited by vasopressin infusion (40 μU/min). This dose of vasopressin, given alone, had no effect on sodium excretion. Vasopressin in common with angiotensin and other vasoactive agents has been shown to inhibit renin secretion (Vandongen 1975).

Summary and Conclusions

Studies on the role of cyclic AMP in the renal action of vasopressin have been extended during the year. Attempts have been made to characterise the membrane receptor for vasopressin and to locate the cell site of the enzymes involved in the response. Doubt has been cast on the belief that vasopressin acts on the distal tubule in some species as vasopressin was unable to stimulate adenyl cyclase in the rabbit distal tubule. As with the amphibian membranes, it appears that microtubules are involved in the vasopressin-induced changes in water permeability in the nephron. In addition to the effects on water permeability, the suggestion has again been raised that vasopressin may affect sodium transport in the kidney.

Chapter 12

VASOPRESSIN AND THE CARDIOVASCULAR SYSTEM

"So the Bellman would cry: and the crew would reply
They are merely conventional signs!"

The pressor effect was the first reported biological activity of vasopressin (Oliver and Schafer, 1895). The hormone produces widespread vasoconstriction although the response through the body is not uniform, some vascular beds being more sensitive than others. Discordant results have been produced on the regional effects of vasopressin, but this may be due to the dose used and the background status of the preparation. It is generally accepted that vasopressin has a peculiar affinity for the skin vessels. The vascular bed of the splanchnic region is another area in which it is claimed that the action of vasopressin is more or less selective. Some exceptions to the rule of general vasoconstriction are said to be the absence of active vasoconstriction in the lungs and possible vasodilation in the liver and kidney. As far as the microcirculation is concerned it seems that the effect is different from that produced by other vasoconstrictor agents. It is suggested that the gradient of reactivity to vasopressin progresses from the venular to the arterial side. For many reasons, including these differences in action, it is improbable that the circulatory action of vasopressin is mediated by other vasoactive substances. There is also evidence to suggest that cAMP is not an intermediate in the response as it is in the kidney. It now appears that vasopressin induces depolarisation of the membrane of vascular smooth muscle, but few studies have been carried out on the excitation contraction mechanism. It is known, however, that high intracellular K^+ and Mg^{++} and low Na^+ increase the vasoconstrictor action of vasopressin.

The vasoconstrictor effects are also associated with changes in cardiac output. There is a fall in heart rate which may be reflexly produced by the increase in blood pressure, although there is evidence of a direct slowing effect on the heart and, in addition, evidence of inhibition of myocardial contractility.

Although it was felt that the action of vasopressin on the cardiovascular system was not of physiological significance, it is now believed that it may be the case. Studies on cardiovascular responses may also be important because of the clinical use of the hormone. As mentioned in Chapter 18, fairly high doses may be used therapeutically.

Action on Arteriolar Smooth Muscle

Recent studies on the action of vasopressin on the cardiovascular system have concentrated on the response of preparations of certain blood vessels and on regional effects of the hormone.

As indicated, the mechanism whereby vasopressin produces contraction of smooth muscle in blood vessels is not well understood. Indeed, smooth muscle on the whole has been relatively neglected. One clue which, if pursued, might throw light on the problem is that of the potentiating effect of Mg^{++}. Altura (1975 a,b,) has taken up the challenge. The suggestion has been made that Mg^{++} acts by potentiating the binding of hormones to the receptors (Somlyo & Somlyo, 1970). Altura's evidence confirms this and also implicates other mechanisms. He prepared helically-cut aortic strips, suspended them isometrically in an organ bath under a tension of 1.5g. He then prepared a cumulative series of log dose response curves at different concentrations of magnesium for nine analogues of vasopressin. The response metameter was taken to be the per cent of maximal isometric contraction achieved at each dose. Magnesium did increase the affinity of the molecules used, as demonstrated by a decrease in the concentration of neurohypophysial hormone (or analogue) to produce 50% of maximum contraction (ED_{50}). The values of ED_{50} for AVP in the two papers quoted above are not, however, the same.

If Mg^{++} were acting solely to alter the receptor binding of neurohypophysial hormones one would expect to see a parallel movement of curves down the log dose. This was not found to be the case. The dose response curves were steepened and the contractile responses were differentially affected. This would suggest that Mg^{++} acts on sites other than the receptors. This could be through competition with Ca^{++} for various intracellular sites so that more Ca^{++} is released for reaction with actomyosin. Alternatively, the actomyosin could be activated directly in the presence of Mg^{++}.

The analogues used were substituted in positions 1, 2, 3 and/or 8. Their actions were not affected equally by Mg^{++}. It was observed that the basicity of the residue at position 8 and the length of the side chain were important in the potentiation by Mg^{++}. The ED_{50} of oxytocin and (3 leu, 8 Orn) vasopressin was not affected by magnesium, suggesting that the aromatic group of AVP in position 3 was important in the interaction of the peptide with smooth muscle. Altura further suggested that his results indicated that the effect of Mg^{++} depended on the potency of the analogues causing vasoconstriction.

In addition to these investigations on the Mg^{++} - neurohypophysial hormone interactions, Altura (1975c) has studied the effect of steroids on the arteriolar response to vasopressin. He developed the concept that sex hormones may play a role in the control of peripheral blood flow and the reactivity of arteriolar smooth muscle. In these studies the responses of the arterioles of the mesentery were perused by microscopic observation. The ED_{50} in female animals for AVP, AVT and oxytocin was significantly lower than in the male and the entire dose response was shifted to the left. Pretreatment of male rats with oestrogen produced a similar enhancement in the neurohypophysial hormone action. Oestrogen produced a similar shift of dose response curves for catecholamines, but not for dopamine, serotonin or angiotensin. These sex-linked responses thus appear to be specific for neurohypophysial hormones and certain α-adrenergic stimulators. Oestrogen is well known to have membrane effects on uterine muscle and other tissues and could well bring about similar changes in arterial smooth muscle.

Oestrogen is not the only steroid to affect the response of arterial smooth muscle to vasopressin. It has been shown by Darke (1975) that glucocorticoids may have the same effect. He observed the effect of dexamethasone on the changes in diameter in the arterioles of the meso-appendix of the rat following application of vasopressin. In five of eleven such preparations there was enhanced pressor activity to what must be considered as large doses of vasopressin (6 - 12 U/ml). Catecholamines produced a similar effect and it has been suggested that the response is mediated via inhibition of catechol-o-methyl transferase. The work of Darke indicates that this is not the underlying mechanism. There is, however, some difficulty in interpreting the results as Altura, Altura & Hershey, (1974) have shown that hydrocortisone and methyl prednisolone inhibit changes produced by vasopressin.

Action of Vasopressin on Intrarenal Flow Distribution

It has been suggested that in addition to enhancing water reabsorption in the kidney vasopressin may also act through redistribution of blood flow through the kidney. This possibility has been re-examined by Morgan, Akatsuka, Wilson, Moran and Sizemore, (1975) who used xenon washout techniques to measure renal blood flow and flow distribution during infusions of vasopressin sufficient to produce circulating concentrations of 2 - 64 μU/ml in lightly anaesthetised dogs. They were able to show changes at the lowest level of infusion. The redistribution of flow and changes in the relative volume of tissue perfused suggest regional variations in vascular sensitivity. There is no indication as to whether vasopressin levels were measured. If no such determinations were made then it is possible that the circulating concentration was higher than estimated as hydration would probably not suppress endogenous release of the hormone in lightly anaesthetised animals.

Regional Vasoconstrictor Effects of Vasopressin

Observation of the regional effects of vasopressin suggested that the hormone may have a role in certain situations such as haemorrhagic shock. This possibility was raised again by Rocha e Silva and Rosenberg (1969), and McNeill, Stark and Greenway (1970) and subsequent work has tended to confirm it. Errington and Rocha e Silva (1974), making a study on the mechanisms of irreversible shock and possible treatment, showed accompanying lesions in the areas supplied by the mesenteric, hepatic and renal arteries. This is a result of the ischaemic anoxia and subsequent stagnant anoxia, produced by the vasoconstriction. Dogs with experimental diabetes insipidus, although developing haemorrhagic shock when 35ml blood per kg were removed for 4½h, maintained a relatively high cardiac output and peripheral vascular conductance. Furthermore, all six dogs survived a three day observation period whereas all the control dogs died within 24h of retransfusion. Dogs treated with BPP_{aa}, which blocks the conversion of angiotensin I to angiotensin II, also survived the control period. It is apparent therefore, that the most important vascular effects in shock are on the mesenteric bed and that the action of vasopressin contributes to this effect. Apart from the direct action of vasopressin, the peptide would also potentiate the vasoconstrictor effect of circulating catecholamines. It is possible also that angiotensin II enhances vasopressin release.

Vasopressin and the renin angiotensin system have been postulated to have a role in causing intestinal vasoconstriction following small changes in blood volume. McNeill (1974) has researched into changes in intestinal resistance pursuant on volume depletion induced by the diuretic agents: frusemide, ethacrynic acid and chlorothiazide. Administration of these agents to pentobarbitone anaesthetised cats produced intestinal vasoconstriction. This was ascribed to the accompanying volume depletion as nephrectomy or replacement of volume equal to the urinary losses prevented the response following frusemide. The renin angiotensin system and vasopressin were said to be involved as the vasoconstrictor response was retained either after intestinal denervation, adrenalectomy, hypophysectomy or after intestinal denervation, adrenalectomy and administration of SQ 20881, an inhibitor of the angiotensin-converting enzyme. Hypophysectomy and treatment with SQ 20881 completely abolished the response. It was surprising in these studies that hypophysectomy did not greatly alter urine flow and, as the author himself comments, that the diuresis in hypophysectomised and adrenalectomised animals was similar to that in the control preparations. It was a pity that estimates of plasma vasopressin could not have been made in the animals with intact pituitaries. After such heroic surgery, one would expect vasopressin to be much elevated and it would have been of interest to see what further rises volume depletion could have caused. Both Rocha e Silva and McNeill treated hypophysectomy as if only vasopressin were affected. One cannot, of course, rule out the effect of oxytocin or any of the anterior pituitary hormones.

Schmid, Abboud, Wendling, Ramberg, Mark, Heistad and Eckstein (1974) have produced further evidence of the varying regional response to vasopressin. They observed the subdivisional vascular responses to infused vasopressin in anaesthetised dogs pretreated with hexamethonium bromide to inhibit cardiovascular reflexes. Electromagnetic flow meters were used to measure flow to the iliac bed, the mesentery and the kidney. Heart rate, cardiac output, and brachial arterial, right atrial and portal venous pressures were also monitored. They found that the iliac bed appeared most sensitive to vasopressin. Since this bed comprises largely skin and muscle they performed further experiments to distinguish between the effects on the gracilis muscle and the hind paw which contains predominantly cutaneous resistance vessels. They found that the muscle vasculature was very sensitive, responding to 28 μU/ml. Increases of this order would be found in some pathophysiological states, but would not under normal conditions. Vasopressin concentrations were measured in these studies by bioassay. The basal levels in these studies were found to be 50 $\pm$ 15 μU/ml (SEM, n = 5). In view of the reported sensitivity of the muscle vessels, it is unfortunate that baseline levels were so high. One suspects that other changes may have been masked. Significant vasoconstriction in the whole iliac bed was produced by a concentration of 144 μU/ml, but this was still more sensitive than the mesentery responding to 215 μU/ml. It was further shown that intravenous infusions caused a marked redistribution of blood from the hind limb, but not from the mesentery and kidney. In fact with the low infusion, producing an increase in vasopressin of 60 μU/ml there was an elevated renal blood flow, indicating redistribution of cardiac output to the kidney. The relative sensitivity of the different vascular beds would seem to be (in order of decreasing sensitivity) muscle, mesentery, kidney.

Summary

The studies described suggest that vasopressin is active on blood vessels in fairly low concentrations. Further vasopressin can act to redistribute circulating blood volume. It is, therefore, likely that vasopressin exerts an effect on the cardiovascular system in the absence of a measurable change in blood pressure. The significance of the cardiovascular responses to vasopressin may, as a result, have been underestimated in the past.

Chapter 13

METABOLIC AND OTHER ACTIONS OF VASOPRESSIN

"It had learnt in ten minutes far more
Than all books
Would have taught it in seventy years."

It is commonplace that as study of a given hormone progresses so the spectrum of its known activity widens. This has not been as true for vasopressin as for some other hormones. Most attention has centred on the antidiuretic and smooth muscle actions of vasopressin. Apart from observations on the influence of neurohypophysial hormones on adenohypophysial function the only other comprehensive studies have been on the metabolic effects of hormones. Although the data obtained by various workers is not consistent and although there are discrepancies between *in vivo* and *in vitro* effects, in general it seems that arginine and lysine vasopressin, if given in the appropriate quantities can produce hyperglycaemia. It has also been reported that vasopressin given to dogs in a dose of 0.01-1.0 IU/kg body weight produces a fall in the free fatty acid concentration in the plasma (Mirsky, 1963) although an increase is produced by subcutaneous injections in the rabbit. The underlying mechanism of these changes and their physiological significance is not clear.

Possible New Roles for Vasopressin

During the past few years some most interesting topics have been pursued. First, there is the possible glycogenolytic activity of vasopressin which could account for the hyperglycaemia response previously reported and, second, there is the possible role of hormone in the acquisition of conditioned reflexes. An abundance of evidence has recently accumulated in support of this second hypothesis, first adumbrated by De Wied and his colleagues. Other possible actions of vasopressin have been reported during the year.

Hepatic Action of Vasopressin

It has been shown that vasopressin, at concentrations producing cardiovascular responses, and within the range recorded after haemorrhage, stimulates glycogen breakdown and gluconeogenesis in the intact rat (Hems and Whitton 1973). Kirk and Hems (1974) have now set out to elucidate the mechanism responsible for the hepatic action of vasopressin. It would seem likely that cyclic AMP (cAMP) participates as it is known to be involved in the renal response to vasopressin (see Chapter 11). Furthermore glucagon and adrenalin are said to produce their catabolic effects through the action of this nucleotide. They followed the changes in the hepatic concentration of cAMP after the administration of vasopressin to intact rats, and the appearance of cAMP in the effluent from the perfused liver. Vasopressin given in doses sufficient to produce an increase in hepatic glucose output, similar to that seen with adrenalin, produced no change in the concentration of cAMP either in the liver or in the effluent. However they were able to demonstrate an increase in cAMP in response to adrenalin and glucagon. This is consistent with the findings that vasopressin has no effect on hepatic adenyl cyclase. It appears therefore that vasopressin is unique in that cAMP is not involved in the glycogenolytic action. Hems, Whitton and Gary (1975) have suggested that the glycogenolysis produced by vasopressin could result from the hypoxia produced as a result of the vasoconstriction of gut vessels.

Further evidence that AVP causes glycogen breakdown via a novel mechanism comes from the work of Keppens and Wulf (1974, 1975). They believe that the hepatic effect of vasopressin is due to activation of glycogen phosphorylase, the rate-limiting enzyme in glycogen degradation, but that it exerts this effect in a different manner from glucagon and noradrenalin. These two hormones, via cAMP, activate protein kinase which leads to conversion of glycogen phosphorylase b to a. Keppens and Wulf conducted their experiments on pentobarbitone anaesthetised, fed rats, taking liver biopsies for estimation of protein kinase and glycogen phosphorylase after the injection of vasopressin. They were able to demonstrate marked increases in phosphorylase and protein kinase activity after glucagon, but following vasopressin administration they observed an increase in phosphorylase activity, but there was no change in protein kinase activity.

Vasopressin and Lipolysis

As already indicated vasopressin has been said to have an effect on fat metabolism, causing the release of free fatty acids from adipose tissue in rabbit and guinea pig, but not pig, rat and dog. Bartsokas, Polychronopoulou - Trichopolou, Kouvelas, Charissiadou, Valsamakis and Kalaitzidou (1975) have taken up this problem. They report that LVP did not produce an increase in free fatty acids in man and the rat.

Furthermore the hormone had no effect on adenyl cyclase activity in the rat epididymal fat pad.

Raij, Harkonen, Mulder and Adlercreutz (1975) have also studied the possible lipolytic action of vasopressin. They gave intravenous doses of 20 and 200 μg at which levels there were increases in free fatty acid concentrations. The authors believe that the C-terminal tripeptide exerted its lipolytic effect directly on the fat cells. They furthermore suggested that the lipolytic action of vasopressin itself could be exerted by this sequence of the octapeptide or by the tripeptide produced. It should be noted however that 20 μg of the tripeptide represents the equivalent of a very large injection of vasopressin (about 30 IU) so that this action is of doubtful physiological significance.

Hems et al (1975) have looked at hormonal control of plasma lipid concentration in the rat. They noted, after vasopressin administration, an initial decrease in plasma free fatty acid concentration accompanying the rise in plasma glucose. At 15 minutes the plasma free fatty acid had begun to rise and the glucose concentration to fall. They suggest that these changes in plasma lipid are secondary to the shifts in plasma glucose concentration and the resultant effect on insulin secretion.

Vasopressin and Memory

A fascinating story currently unfolding is that concerning the effect of vasopressin on the memory processes in the rat. In many of these studies, the extinction of learnt passive and active avoidance behaviour has been observed. The studies on passive avoidance depend on the innate preference of the rat for darkness as opposed to light. The animals are pretrained to enter a dark box and on the final trial, they are given a foot shock on entry into the box; the latency of entering the dark box is then followed in a series of further trials. A shuttle box was used to study the active avoidance response. The rats were trained to avoid an unconditioned stimulus, an electric floor shock, by jumping onto a pole in the centre of the apparatus. The unconditioned stimulus was applied if the avoidance response did not occur within five seconds of the conditioned stimulus which was in this case a light in the top of the box. There is a body of evidence to show that vasopressin effects the behavioural response of rats in this system. Bohus, Ader and de Wied (1971) found that administration of lysine vasopressin (LVP) resulted in resistance to extinction of the avoidance behaviour, provided it was given at a certain point in the training of the animal. It was effective on active avoidance behaviour if given one hour before the final acquisition conditioning session but not six hours before. Similar observations were made for the extinction of passive avoidance behaviour. This and much other work has been summarised in three reviews, by De

Wied and his colleagues (De Wied, 1973; De Wied, Bohus and Van Wimersma–Greidanus, 1974; Van Wimersma-Greidanus, Bohus and De Wied, 1975).

As long ago as 1965, De Wied showed that removal of the posterior pituitary lobe led to more rapid extinction of the shuttle box avoidance response. The Brattleboro rat, with hereditary diabetes insipidus (DI) (see Chapter 17), would, of course, provide an excellent system for testing the effect of vasopressin on memory. De Wied, Bohus and Van Wimersma-Greidanus (1974) have therefore studied the period of retention latency following the passive avoidance in homozygous DI rats (i.e. those with the syndrome) and heterozygous animals. The heterozygous rats showed passive avoidance behaviour and the retention tendency increased with the intensity of the shock. The homozygous animals on the other hand exhibited no passive avoidance behavious. Thus, lack of AVP seems to affect memory adversely in these rats. The responses of the homozygous rats could be brought in line with those of their heterozygous companions by a subcutaneous injection of 1μg vasopressin. This effect did not appear to be due to a difference in the sensitivities to shock of the two groups of rats, neither did it appear to be a result of the state of water balance. Desglycinamide lysine vasopressin (DG-LVP), which has little antidiuretic or, indeed, pressor activity, restores the memory deficit in DI rats.

The analogue DG-LVP has also been shown to be effective in antagonizing CO_2 -induced retrograde anmesia in rats (Rigter, van Riezen and De Wied, 1974). The test used was the "step through" passive avoidance situation. After the acquisition trial the animals were exposed to a CO_2 atmosphere which contained no oxygen and then given a test trial. DG-LVP was effective in preserving conditioning if given one hour prior to the acquisition or test trial. This would indicate that LVP facilitates the consolidation process, or protects the memory consolidation from the adverse effects of CO_2 treatment. The fact that the vasopressin analogue was effective when given after the acquisition trial, just before the test trial, also suggests that DG-LVP reverses the effects of CO_2–induced amnesia or promotes the memory retrieval.

Further proof for the hypothesis of De Wied and his colleagues has come from the use of a recently available tool, namely a specific antiserum to vasopressin. If vasopressin is necessary for the retention of certain types of learnt behaviour, then presumably inactivation of the natural hormone with antiserum should impair the learning process; Van Wimersma–Greidanus and Bohus and De Wied, 1975; Van Wimersma–Greidanus, Dogteram and De Wied (1975) have adopted this technique. They administered the antiserum both intravenously and intra-cisternally, as it had been previously shown that vasopressin analogues have a greater effect on behavioural responses if applied within the central nervous system or the cerebrospinal fluid. Intraventricular administration of anti-vasopressin serum (1μ1) antiserum raised against thyroglobulin-coupled AVP inhibited memory expression in rats. Oxytocin antiserum was ineffective. Intravenous administration was ineffective, even when one hundred times as much was given as intracisternally. It was felt that the amount of antiserum used virtually removed all vasopressin from the circulation and, in fact, no vasopressin could be demonstrated in the urine of these rats. In view of these results it must be surmised that vasopressin exerts its behavioural effects via the CSF. As mentioned in Chapter 2, there is a pathway by which neurohypophysial hormones can reach the CSF and neurophysin has already been detected in the CSF. It appears that the memory process, rather than learning, is affected as no alteration was seen in the passive avoidance behaviour of the rats treated with antiserum if they were tested less than one hour after the learning trial. The deficiency only became apparent on tests carried out 24 and 48 hours later.

Another fact to emerge from the studies of De Wied is that there is no generalisation, i.e. no transfer of the effect of vasopressin from one behavioural situation to another. There is a close temporal relationship between the administration of vasopressin and the altered behavioural response. Vasopressin is released in response to a number of specific stimuli (see Chapter 9) but also in response to the less well defined stimulus of 'stress'. The value of vasopressin release under these conditions is not clear, but could lie in its role in fixing behavioural responses in stressful situations. This would allow selective retention of information and corresponding behaviour patterns. Those learnt under adverse conditions and possibly of more value to the organism would be more likely to be remembered. Here, though, one is entering the realms of conjecture. It appears that vasopressin is first released into the CSF and thereafter exerts its effect on memory. There is virtually no information available as to how the peptide could bring about these changes. Studies with analogues, as used in other situations could be of value in identifying the receptor site.

Flexner, Flexner, Hoffman and Walter (1975) have reported on some preliminary observations on this topic, using analogues and fragments of neurohypophysial hormones. They studied the amnesic affects of puromycin treatment and found that they could be reduced by the long acting analogues [tri-Gly] LVP and 1 - deamino - 8 - D - Arg] AVP. Fragments with the amino acid sequence of the terminal tripeptide of LVP had a similar effect whereas the terminal tripeptide of oxytocin was effective.

In many of these studies DeWied and his colleagues have used one trial passive avoidance situations. Garrud (1975) has been able to confirm the effect of LVP on behaviour in investigations under continuing punishment conditions - the punishment-induced suppression of a lever-holding response. Rats were deprived of food and then trained to obtain food as a reward if they pressed down a lever for eight seconds. Once they had been trained to complete the manoeuvre, an electric shock was delivered at eight seconds with the food. Administration of LVP prolonged the time between the response and increased the efficiency expressed as the ratio of the number of reinforced holds, (i.e. those lasting longer than 8 seconds), to the total number of holds.

Neurohypophysial Hormones as Prohormones

Vasopressin is known to cause the release of ACTH and for some time was considered to play a physiological role in ACTH release. Although this view is no longer held, there is considerable evidence that fragments of neurohypophysial hormones exert activity on the pituitary in addition to the action on the central nervous system, already described. Walter (1974) has reviewed this subject and proposed that neurohypophysial hormones, which are probably derived from precursors of high molecular weight, could themselves act as precursors for a further set of hormonal factors comprising three to five amino acids, which act on the central nervous system. Thus, the terminal tripeptide of oxytocin, Proc-Leu-Gly NA_2, inhibits the release of MSH (Celis, Taleisnik and Walter, 1971) and pressinoic acid has potent ACTH releasing activity (Saffran, Pearlmutter, Rapino and Upton, 1972).

It has been suggested that oxytocin might also be involved in the release of prolactin. Forsling, Reinhardt and Himmler, (1974) therefore investigated the relationship of the release of neurohypophysial hormones to prolactin release during milking. They were able to demonstrate the release of oxytocin and vasopressin during milking but there appeared to be no direct relationship with prolactin release. However, the highest prolactin concentration was only reached after the final oxytocin peak so that the possibility cannot be excluded that oxytocin acts as a primer for prolactin release.

Vaughan, Reiter, McKinney and Vaughan (1974) have looked at the action of arginine vasotocin (AVT) a naturally occurring analogue of vasopressin found in the pineal gland (Rosenbloom and Fisher, 1975). They found that AVT, when injected into immature male Swiss Webster mice and hamsters, retarded growth of the ventral prostate and accessory sex organs. It is possible therefore that oxytocin acts on the central nervous system to affect synthesis or release of gonadotrophins. Alternatively, since the terminal tripeptide of AVT, Pro - Arg - Gly NH_2, has the same amino acids as the terminal peptide of luteinising hormone releasing hormone (LHRH), it is possible that AVT or its degradation products block the binding of LHRH to its receptor sites.

There is considerable evidence that vasopressin is not normally involved in the release of ACTH and that there is a specific corticotrophin releasing factor CRF. Since the posterior pituitary appears to be the main source of CRF, Fehm, Voigt and Lang (1975) have attempted to distinguish, on the basis of bioassay, between the CRF-like activity of vasopressin and CRF. Bioassay was carried out using isolated pituitary cells, the ACTH release being determined by radioimmunoassay. The nature of the dose response curves obtained with the pure peptides and extracts of the median eminence or the posterior pituitary indicated that the CRF activity of these extracts was not due to contamination with vasopressin.

Vasopressin and Blood Factors

Another process on which vasopressin is said to act is fibrinolysis (Schneck and Van Kaulla 1961; Mannucci, Perego and Barbi 1972). In fairly high concentration it appears to increase the concentration of plasminogen activator in plasma. Cash, Gader and da Costa (1974) report that the analogue (DDAVP) is particularly effective in this respect, producing a sustained response without side effects when infused into healthy volunteers. These observations are not only of pure academic interest as these peptides could be used in fibrinolytic therapy. Furthermore, as discussed in Chapters 3 and 18, vasopressin may be used in treatment in many conditions. It can, for example, be used to control bleeding in the gastrointestinal tract, or to improve the efficiency of local anaesthetics, particularly in dental work. If vasopressin is used in selective intra-arterial infusion to control bleeding from lesions such as oesophageal varices, it is given in fairly high concentrations and the fibrinolysis which may be produced is undesirable. It is also interesting to speculate on the effect of the high concentrations of vasopressin, which have been reported to occur following surgery.

The mechanism whereby hormones exert their effect on plasminogen activator is unknown but not surprisingly a role has been ascribed to cyclic AMP. Mannucci, Pareti and Barbi (1974) were unable to find evidence to support the suggestion that cyclic AMP is the second messenger for the increase in plasminogen activity of the blood which is produced by vasopressin infusion in man. The action of vasopressin on fibrinolysis was not potentiated by theophylline; it was not modified by cyclic AMP, nor by its dibutyryl analogue.

Macfarlane and Mills (1975) have reported that vasopressin in fairly high concentrations (100 mU/ml) can induce primary aggregation of human platelets. Their investigations show that this occurs by a mechanism independent of extracellular ADP.

Further Actions of Vasopressin

Another action reported to occur at physiological concentrations is that on resting gastro-oesophageal sphincter pressure. Infusion at relatively low doses of vasopressin (50 μU/kg/min) in normal subjects produced a significant increase in this pressure (Boesby and Pederson 1974). It seems therefore that vasopressin is involved in the autoregulation of the gastrointestinal tract. Abdominal receptors could be involved in the response.

Changes suggestive of vasopressin involvement, in some respects allied to that in the kidney, are those in aqueous humour outflow in the rabbit. Cole and Nagasubramamian (1973) proposed that intraocular pressure could be maintained under conditions of changing body hydration through the action of vasopressin, the hormone tending to increase aqueous humour formation. The experiments of Nagasubramanian (1974) do not support this hypothesis. Rather they illustrate that, in the rabbit, vasopressin is not likely to affect outflow and any effect that there might be would be to lower intraocular pressure rather than increase it.

Perris and Hunt (1975) have produced some results which suggest that vasopressin released during haemorrhage may act not only to produce vasoconstriction, but to stimulate ,formation of blood cells. Bone marrow mitotic activity in rats has been shown to surge four hours after bleeding - an effect not observed following hypophysectomy, or in the rat with hereditary diabetes insipidus. Furthermore vasopressin was shown to stimulate bone marrow proliferation *in vivo* and *in vitro*.

Davis and Withrington (1975) were able to show that, in addition to the vasoconstrictor action in the blood vessels of the spleen, vasopressin (10 mU given as a close arterial injection) caused contraction of the smooth muscle of the splenic capsule. It is unlikely that this response is of any great physiological significance as in those conditions where relatively large amounts of vasopressin would be released, the capsule would be maximally contracted under the influence of sympathetic activity and circulating catecholamines.

Summary and Conclusions

During the year many possible actions of vasopressin have been investigated. Two particularly interesting subjects which have been studied in detail are the memory-enhancing action and the glycogenolytic action. A considerable body of evidence has accumulated which indicates that vasopressin limits extinction of learnt, passive and active avoidance responses in the rat. This could allow responses learnt under stressful conditions to be better remembered. The second action, that on glycogen breakdown, has been demonstrated both *in vitro* and *in vivo* and could even be supposed to play a role in fluid balance since a certain amount of water is released on glycogen breakdown.

Chapter 14

METABOLISM OF VASOPRESSIN

"You boil it in sawdust: you salt it in glue:
You condense it with locusts and tape:"

In order to comprehend fully the patterns of release and mechanism of action of a hormone, knowledge of the rate and manner of *in vivo* destruction is necessary. Many studies have been performed on this aspect of vasopressin biochemistry, which have been critically and extensively reviewed by Lauson (1974), who discusses the clearance from plasma and inactivation in various organs and isolated tissues. Metabolism depends to a degree on the nature of the circulating hormone. Considerable controversy has surrounded this point, but it would appear that the majority circulates in the unbound form. Estimates of half-time in plasma again show considerable variation, but in all species studied it is relatively short. The half-time of disappearance from the circulation (t½) in man has been shown to be 5.6 min using bioassay measurements (Fabian, Forsling, Jones and Pryor, 1969) and 7.3 min by radioimmunoassay (Beardwell, 1971). Estimates have been made from the decay curve following either an injection or an infusion of vasopressin. As Lauson points out, there are disadvantages to both techniques as they have been performed to date. Interpretation of results following injection is clouded by loss of hormone from the plasma by diffusion. The reverse is true if an infusion is used; hormone diffuses back into the plasma at varying rates after the infusion is stopped. Lauson (1974) suggests the use of a two compartment or three compartment model in the analysis of data from such investigations.

Relatively little destruction of vasopressin occurs in the plasma. The major site of clearance is the kidney, although only a small proportion of the peptide, approximately 10% of an administered dose appears in the urine in the biologically active form. The liver also contributes to the removal of the hormone from the circulation.

It has been claimed that several enzyme pathways are involved in the destruction of neurohypophysial hormones. Surprisingly extensive research has been performed on the amino peptidases which successively attack the peptide bonds from the amino terminal after prior destruction of the disulphide bond. It appears that this type of attack might not be significant in the destruction of AVP. Attack from the C terminal end is probably more important and trypsin–like and chymotrypsin-like pathways have been identified in extracts of several tissues, including kidney.

Clearance of Vasopressin from Plasma

Few studies on the metabolism of AVP have been published during the year. Estimates of t½ have been made both by bioassay and radioimmunoassay. As indicated in chapter 4, it is possible that in this situation there is dissociation of the results obtained by the two assay methods. Forsling, Boyd and Chard (1971) reported this phenomenon with oxytocin. The results depend on the particular antiserum used. In an attempt to find a possible explanation for the observation that vasopressin is diuretic rather than antidiuretic in some circumstances, Yesberg, Henderson and Budtz-Olsen (1975) made estimates for AVP in Merino sheep. They calculated the rate of disappearance of antidiuretic activity from plasma after infusion of vasopressin for 60 min. They report a t½ of 4 min, clearance of 6.9 ml/Kg/min and a volume of distribution of 48 ml/Kg. These values are not greatly different from other observations on animals of a similar size and could not account for the difference in action. Alexander, Britton and Forsling (1976), for example, found a t½ of 6.0 min and clearance of 11.4 ml/Kg/min in sheep of the Welsh Mountain breed.

Burguburu and Geelen (1974) measured the t½ of LVP in 10 subjects using radioimmunoassay and quote a value of 12.7 $\pm$ 0.47 min. They described an exponential fall of LVP concentration in the blood, but only followed the disappearance for 10 min. Fabian et al (1969) gave estimates of a shorter half-time. Both these studies employed LVP and it has been reported that t½ for LVP is shorter in some species than that for AVP; Fabian et al made no such finding in man.

Enzyme Inactivation of Vasopressin in the Kidney

Inactivation of vasopressin by homogenates and extracts of kidney have been shown by many investigators. For example, Borth, Hutter, Pliska and Sorm (1969) have shown that both soluble and particulate fractions of porcine kidney were able to destroy the antidiuretic activity of both lysine and arginine vasopressin. Walter and Shlank (1975) have followed the enzyme inactivation of arginine vasopressin by rat kidney supernatant fluid. They compared the mode of inactivation with that of oxytocin. The renal enzymes were prepared by homogenizing freshly excised kidney in phosphate buffer (pH 6.8) and then centrifuging at 150,000g at 4°C for 1h. The clear supernatant was used in the enzyme studies. Destruction of [9-^{14}C-1-Glycinamide] vasopressin was followed and the degradation products separated and identified with chromato-electrophoresis. The major pathway of inactivation was cleavage of the Pro-Arg bond with the release of Arg (^{14}C) Gly-NH_2. Small amounts of (^{14}C) Gly-NH_2 were also found but it was felt that this was not released directly from the hormone, but formed by secondary cleavage of Arg-Gly-NH_2. Cleavage of the Pro-Leu bond of oxytocin probably occurred at a similar rate to the cleavage of Pro-Arg bond in vasopressin. The more rapid overall destruction of oxytocin was attributed to the action of a chymotrypsin-like enzyme which released Gly-NH_2 from the hormone. Direct release of Gly-NH_2 from vasopressin was slower and seemed to be of minor importance. The relatively slower inactivation of vasopressin could in part account for the relatively higher proportion of biologically active vasopressin, compared with oxytocin, said to be excreted in the urine.

The observation that there are in the kidney enzymes capable of destroying vasopressin, is not surprising as polypeptide hormones are commonly seen to be inactivated in their target organs. It is possible that enzymes within the vicinity of the site of action of vasopressin might serve to regulate the local, and hence the active, concentration of vasopressin in addition to clearing it. Nardacci, Mukhopadhyay and Compbell(1975) therefore investigated the possibility of enzymic activity associated with renal plasma membranes. These were prepared by making homogenates of porcine medulla and carrying out successive centrifugations, the pellet obtained at 35,000 being used in these studies. The plasma membranes thus prepared were found to destroy progressively the activity of vasopressin as determined by the pressor assay. The time course of inactivation for this particular system and in the conditions used was greater than that for the preparation by Walter and Shlank, (1975). In this case 10% of the biological activity remained after 120 min. The soluble preparation by Walter in the circumstances used, destroyed all the vasopressin in 20 min.

Nardacci and his associates performed partial purification of the peptidase by Lubrol Px solubilisation of the membranes and subsequent DEAE cellulose hydroxyapatite and 8% agarose column chromatography. They achieved an 83–fold purification. The groups released from the hormone through the activity of this peptidase were identified using 2,4,6 trinitrobenzene sulphuric acid. Thin layer chromatography showed that the main product of hydrolysis was glycinamide. Thus a chymotrypsin-like enzyme was involved, which was subsequently shown to be inhibited strongly by Ca^{++} and to a lesser degree by Mg^{++}. The molecular weight of the peptidase was estimated according to the method of Andrews (1964) using an 8% agarose column. One drawback of these investigations was the high concentration of vasopressin used (3×10^{-4}M). The authors hoped that development of adenylate-antidiuretic hormone sensitive assays would allow investigations in using vasopressin in the range 10^{-6} - 10^{-20}M, which would be more 'physiological'.

Peptidase Activity in the Pineal Gland

Enzymes capable of inactivating neurohypophysial hormones have previously been demonstrated in the central nervous system and pituitary gland; and now Reinharz and Vallotton (1974) have demonstrated the presence of a peptidase in the bovine pineal gland. The enzyme appeared to be fairly specific in that it attacked AVP and AVT, but not the neurophysins. Studies using inhibitors indicated that an amino group of the enzyme is involved in the action.

Glutathione-Oxytocin Transhydrogenase Activity in Placenta

Interest in the enzymes of pregnancy, capable of destroying neurohypophysial hormones, has largely centred on oxytocinase found in pregnancy serum. It has also been shown that placental extracts can inactivate oxytocin and vasopressin (Hawker, 1956). This finding has been looked at more extensively by Small and Watkins (1974) using as the enzyme preparation clear placental extracts prepared by homogenisation and centrifugation at 105,000g. This preparation contained glutathione-protein transhydrogenase activity which was relatively specific for oxytocin and vasopressin. Thus the placenta, like the kidney, possesses a system for reducing the disulphide in addition to the proteolytic enzyme system (cystine amino peptidase - see below).

Inactivation by Human Pregnancy Serum

As mentioned, one system capable of degrading AVP which has been extensively studied by many laboratories throughout the world is the oxytocinase-vasopressinase system found in the plasma of pregnant women. Since it makes only a small contribution to the overall clearance of hormones, its physiological significance is not clear. The main action is cleavage between the amino terminal hemi-cystine and the tyrosine. It differs from amino peptidase purified from the liver in that it can additionally break the pentapeptide ring. Despite the numerous studies performed on this system, it still excites interest and Molnarova and Sova (1975) have studied the influence of pH on inactivation of neurohypophysial hormones by human pregnancy serum. They employed polarographic techniques and parallel analysis of free amino acids to monitor the reaction in serum from pregnant and non-pregnant women over the pH range 2.5 to 8. They confirmed that the optimum pH range was 5.5 to 8, but found a notable, though less pronounced, optimum at pH 3 to 4.5. The authors hypothesised the existence of iso enzymes of oxytocinase and probable presence of several peptidases with overlapping specificity.

Summary

Relatively few studies on the metabolism of vasopressin have appeared during the year. Observations have confirmed the short half-time of the peptide in plasma and have indicated that the main mechanism for inactivation is enzymic attack of the tail moiety rather than the pentapeptide ring.

Chapter 15

THE FOETAL NEUROHYPOPHYSIS

"While strange creepy creatures came out of their dens,
And watched them with wondering eyes."

An exciting concept, recently developed, is that the foetus plays a role in the initiation of parturition. This is an attractive hypothesis since the foetus is presumably the best judge of intrauterine conditions and the appropriate time for delivery. Monitoring of the foetal endocrine system during the latter half of gestation, especially in the sheep, has been made possible by using chronically catheterised foetal preparations in combination with sensitive hormone assays.

Striking changes in the concentration of some hormones are seen towards full term, the increase in plasma cortisol being particularly noteworthy. Indeed plasma cortisol in the foetus is now used as an indicator of the time of foetal delivery. This information, taken with many other observations including the fact that foetal hypophysectomy delays parturition, had led to the belief that the foetal pituitary adrenal axis is important in parturition.

The fact that the posterior pituitary is removed when hypophysectomy is performed, makes it possible that foetal neurohypophysial hormones could also play a role. Several studies have therefore been performed on the foetal neurohypophysis. An early observation of interest was the finding by Hoppenstein, Miltenberger and Moran (1968), and Chard, Hudson Edwards and Boyd (1971) that foetal cord blood contains high concentrations of oxytocin and vasopressin. Neurohypophysial hormones have also been demonstrated in fairly high concentrations in the foetal pituitary of the guinea pig (Burton and Forsling,1972); rat (Forsling, 1973) and sheep (Alexander, Britton, Forsling, Nixon and Ratcliffe, 1973; Vizsolyi and Perks, 1969) during the latter half of gestation . A high vasopressin: oxytocin ratio was also noted. Vasopressin has been shown to be readily released in the foetus (Alexander et al 1973; Skowsky, Bashore, Smith and Fisher, 1973). although oxytocin was not.

Foetal Pituitary Content

Perks and Vizsolyi (1974) studied the neurohypophysial peptides in the foetal sheep and fur seals. It has been shown that vasopressin appears earlier in the foetal gland than oxytocin and these authors produced histological evidence that there was indeed an earlier onset of synthesis of vasopressin by the supraoptic nucleus. In addition they were able to show that at mid-term the neurohypophysis contained arginine vasotocin. This peptide was first separated from oxytocin and vasopressin by column chromatography and then identified by its pharmacological actions and amino acid composition. This provides an intriguing example of ontology repeating phylogeny. The content of vasotocin falls towards term, whereas that of vasopressin and oxytocin increases. Froger and Rofti, (1974) showed a rapid increase in the antidiuretic activity in the foetal rabbit neurohypophysis during the last few days before parturition. At day 30 the content was 60mU, but by day 31 it had increased to 125mU. The content, however, fell to 75mU half an hour after birth. Burton and Forsling (1972) reported a similar increase in vasopressin and neurophysin in the guinea pig foetus at birth.

Pearson, Goodman and Sachs, (1975) also found a pronounced increase in the vasopressin and neurophysin content between the 40th and 50th days of gestation in the guinea pig (term being variable but about 64 days). They too found vasopressin and neurophysin were first detectable around day 30 to 35. The amounts of the two peptides present were very small at this stage. There was a gradual increase to day 40, but by day 53 a 100 fold increase in levels. They were able to confirm this increase in synthesis in organ culture of the hypothalamo-neurohypophysial complex (HNC) from the foetal guinea pig. Thus, whereas incorporation of radioactivity into neurophysin or vasopressin could not be detected in preparations from the young foetus, it was clearly demonstrable at day 45. They suggest that this augmentation of vasopressin and neurophysin synthesis is due to the production of a stimulating factor in the foetal hypothalamo-hypophysial system. Evidence for this was provided by studies on cultures of the adult HNC, a preparation used in previous studies and whose characteristics were well known. Incorporation of radioactive label into the adult preparation was elevated in the presence of HNC tissue from a 45 day foetus. A similar stimulation was seen if extracts of foetal hypothalamo-neurohypophysial preparations were added to the adult tissue. Extracts of foetal liver or cerebral cortex were ineffective. These workers are uncertain as to the nature of the factor involved, but preliminary studies suggest that it is a polypeptide with molecular weight probably greater than 5,000.

Release of Vasopressin in the Foetus

Having shown that vasopressin is present in the neurohypophysis and in fairly high levels in the foetus of some species, it is necessary to establish whether the mechanisms for release are functional and to identify the factors involved, before a possible role can be assigned to the foetal hormone.

Skowsky et al (1973), using a sensitive radioimmunoassay, found fairly high resting concentration of vasopressin, suggesting a high basal rate of secretion. Alexander, Britton, Forsling, Nixon and Ratcliffe (1974) found the AVP was below the limit of detection (i.e.$<$ 5 μU/ml) in the plasma of younger foetuses (90-107 days). Pregnancy in the breed of sheep used lasts 147 days. The samples were taken from the acutely exposed foetus, the mother being anaesthetised by spinal administration of procaine. The values reported could, therefore, be higher than the resting levels *in utero*. Foetuses were subsequently subjected to bleeds of 10-15ml at intervals of 15-20mins. since haemorrhage is known to be a potent releaser of vasopressin in the adult. A massive release of hormones ensued when 20% or more of the estimated blood volume had been removed from foetuses of 90–107 days, and even greater concentrations were achieved in the older animals. There was no correlation between foetal and maternal levels suggesting that the placenta is relatively impermeable to vasopressin., The anterior pituitary hormones, growth hormone and adrenocorticotrophin (ACTH) were also studied in this investigation. Foetal ACTH changes were similar to those of AVP; the growth hormone response was less consistent. It appears, therefore, that AVP is readily released from the foetal pituitary, and in considerable quantities, by a stimulus effective in the adult. Haemorrhage, however, is not a very 'physiological' stimulus, but it has been demonstrated that vasopressin is released in response to hypoxia which is a more likely occurrence *in utero*.

Having shown that fairly high concentrations of AVP can be reached in the foetal animal Alexander, Bashore, Britton, and Forsling (1974) went on to monitor AVP concentrations in the sheep foetus during the last 18 days of pregnancy. These studies were carried out on the conscious, chronically catheterised preparation. Until the last few days before delivery AVP was undetectable ($\ll$3.5 μU/ml) in the foetus. In the 48h. preceeding delivery the AVP concentrations began to show marked increases, the highest concentration (up to 45 μU/m1) being found at the time of delivery. Vasopressin in the maternal circulation was also low until the last week. The increases then seen, however, were small compared with those in the foetus, being the order of a few microunits. This apparently enhanced vasopressin secretion did not seem to be a result of "stress" associated with catheterisation as high concentrations were found in samples taken from a non-catheterised foetus at the time of delivery. It is, however, impossible to rule out "stress" associated with parturition under experimental conditions. Sheep are not the placid creatures one might imagine.

Action of Foetal Neurohypophysial Hormones

The foetal pituitary thus contains neurohypophysial hormones from an early stage of gestation and it appears that vasopressin circulates in the plasma in measurable quantities especially near term. What then is the role of AVP in the foetal animal, since it need not have a water conserving function as in the adult? The foetal kidneys are little influenced by neurohypophysial hormones, but they could act on other tissues and thereby influence fluid economy. Perks and Vizsolyi (1974) have shown that AVT acted on the isolated amniotic membrane of the guinea pig causing the flow of fluid from mother to foetus to slow or even reverse. As a result it was suggested that AVT and/or AVP are excreted through the foetal kidney, pass into the urine and thence to the amniotic cavity to act on the amnion and thereby maintain amniotic volume.

Bailey, France, Parry and Stanier (1975) have put forward the intriguing suggestion that since the foetus occupies an environment similar in many ways to that of an amphibian, it is possible that AVP acts on the skin and bladder in the foetus. AVP and AVT increased $^3H_20$ fluxes and sodium transport against a gradient in the bladder, although sodium influx through the skin was depressed by AVT. However, very high concentrations of the hormone were used, 5.5 mU/ml AVT and 0.2 U/ml AVP.

The function of increased foetal AVP towards term is again a matter for speculation. Although oxytocin is more effective than AVP in stimulating contraction of the pregnant uterus of the rat, Heller (1974) has shown that oestrodial raises the relative activity of vasopressin to 27% of that of oxytocin. Such a change in the potency might well happen at term when maternal oestrogen levels rise markedly. AVP could also exert an effect through its action on blood vessels for, by reducing placental boood flow, it could interfere with placental hormone production. It could also play a role in causing redistribution of blood flow in the foetus. Finally, it could even act on the umbilical blood vessels. Altura, Malaviya, Reich and Orkin (1972) and Roache (1973) have shown that both AVP and oxytocin are effective in causing contraction of the umbilical vessels. All this, of course, is highly speculative and further studies are needed to elucidate the role of vasopressin, if any, in the foetus.

Summary and Conclusions

The interest in the role of foetal hormones in the onset of parturition has focussed attention on the foetal neurohypophysis. It seems that in a number of species oxytocin, vasopressin and the carrier protein neurophysin are produced quite early in gestation. Although oxytocin is not readily released, vasopressin secretion is stimulated by a number of stimuli shown to be effective in the adult. Vasopressin concentration in the plasma of foetal lambs rises towards full term, but the significance of this increase is not fully understood.

Chapter 16

SYNDROME OF INAPPROPRIATE SECRETION OF ANTIDIURETIC HORMONE

"Come, listen, my men, while I tell you again
The five unmistakable marks."

For most hormones the conditions associated with hypersecretion were characterised early in the history of that particular hormone. This is not the case with vasopressin. The nature of changes to be expected in the presence of elevated vasopressin levels was indicated by Leaf, Bartter, Santos and Wong (1953) who administered Pitressin to a group of control subjects. The syndrome of inappropriate secretion of ADH (SIADH) was first described by Barrter and Schwarz and their colleagues (1967) in patients with bronchial carcinoma. This syndrome is characterised by the production of a relatively concentrated urine, often hypertonic to plasma (Novich, 1975) and continued sodium excretion in the face of marked hyponatraemia, levels of below 110mmol/l being reported. Other features are an increase in extracellular fluid volume, an inability to excrete a water load normally, but otherwise normal renal and adrenal function. Elevated plasma vasopressin has also been demonstrated in some patients. The clinical signs are those of water intoxication. The patient is irritable and drowsy and then follows a period of nausea and vomiting. As the condition progresses neurological symptoms predominate - convulsions, stupor and coma. The condition is improved by fluid restriction.

Although first described in association with cancer, many hundreds of cases associated with a variety of clinical conditions have now been described. It has been shown that with lung cancer, the tumour itself is a source of AVP. In other cases it must be assumed that the hormone is of pituitary origin. This, of course, raises the question of the definition of inappropriate secretion. It is generally taken that the secretion is inappropriate for the plasma osmolality. It could be that it is appropriate for the 'stress' to which the patient has been subjected (see Chapter 9) or the drug regime etc. used. The underlying causes of certain features of the syndrome are as yet unresolved. Thus, the extent of the hyponatraemia cannot generally be accounted for by the degree of overhydration or the sodium loss.

Many reviews have been written on the subject of SIADH. Bartter and Schwarz prepared a comprehensive description for a symposium on antidiuretic hormones published in the American Journal of Medicine (1967). Several reviews have appeared during the year. Rutsky (1975) considers the mechanisms involved in production and secretion of vasopressin and its mode of action. He describes the salient features of the syndrome and the possible forms of therapy raising the point that treatment should be aimed at the underlying disorder as inhibition of vasopressin release is not generally feasible. Scheiner (1975) has written a more lengthy discussion with 180 references. As well as describing normal antidiuretic hormone metabolism, she attempts to clarify the relationship between the hormone and the clinical conditions associated with its excess. Moses and Miller (1974) have summarised knowledge of drug-induced dilutional hyponatraemia. The possible causes of inappropriate secretion of ADH are considered here under a number of headings. A summary is given in table 1 which provides a useful classification for the present discussion.

TABLE 1

Conditions associated with SIADH

(1) Ectopic Production
- Tumours
- Tuberculous tissue

(2) Central Nervous System Diseases
- e.g. Meningitis
- Cerebrovascular Disease

(3) Intrathoracic Processes
- Thoracic Disease
- Other disorders e.g. positive pressure ventilation

(4) Endocrine Disorders

(5) Drugs
- e.g. Diuretics
- Oral hypoglycaemic agents
- Antineoplastic agents

Tumours

Rees and Ratcliffe (1974) have reviewed the subject of ectopic hormone production. It has been suggested that inappropriate vasopressin production could be due to factors other than synthesis by the tumour. There are a number of criteria which must be fulfilled before a hormone can be considered as ectopic in origin. The tumor should be associated with the clinical endocrine syndrome and elevated or inappropriate plasma levels should be seen. There should be a fall in hormone levels, possibly with regression of the clinical syndrome after removal of the tumour, but no such changes after removal of the gland normally producing the hormone. Final proof is given by an arterio-venous hormone gradient across the tumour bed, demonstration of the hormone in the tumour tissue and, if possible, secretion of the hormone by the tumour in culture. Obviously there are many problems in fulfilling these criteria. However, many have been satisfied for AVP. Furthermore, oxytocin and neurophysin have been found in tumours from patients with hyponatraemia. This would suggest that the synthetic processes are similar to those normally producing neurohypophysial peptides.

Vorherr and his colleagues, who have contributed much to our knowledge of the association of vasopressin-like material with malignant tumours, have produced further evidence that malignant tumours contain a vasopressin-like substance even in the absence of SIADH (Vorherr, Vorherr, McConnell, Goldberg, Kornfeld & Jordan, 1974). These studies were made in five patients with malignant tumours; three with bronchial carcinoma (two of whom had no clinical signs of SIADH), one adenocarcinoma of the pancreas and one carcinoma of the uterus. The bronchial carcinoma and the adenocarcinoma all contained antidiuretic activity determined by bioassay in the water-loaded rat anaesthetised with alcohol. This was identified as vasopressin as it could be inactivated with vasopressin antiserum or pregnancy plasma and possessed the appropriate degree of milk-ejecting activity (i.e. 15% of an equivalent quantity of oxytocin). The zone of active tumour growth contained most of the antidiuretic activity. They were also able to demonstrate that these cancer cells suspended in bicarbonate saline could release ADH and that small amounts of ADH were synthesised by the tumour tissue in culture. Measurement of plasma and urinary ADH in one patient showed a modest elevation in circulating ADH from a normal of 0.4-0.6 μU/ml to 2.9 μU/ml. Massive increases in plasma ADH are thus not needed to produce the syndrome. Such small changes in plasma ADH have a marked effect on the kidney and if maintained over a prolonged period of time could produce changes in sodium and water balance. As a result of these studies Vorherr et al suggested that ADH measurement in plasma and more especially in urine could lead to early diagnosis of lung cancer.

SIADH has also been reported in a case of Ewings carcinoma (Zimbler, Robertson, Bartter, Delea and Pomeroy, 1975). The serum sodium fell as low as 117 mmol/l. Vasopressin was also measured, but by radioimmunoassay. When the plasma osmolality was 268 mOsm/Kg, a value of 4.6 pg/ml (1.8μU/ml) was found. Robertson, Mahr, Athar and Sinha (1973) have reported that with this assay they would normally expect to find a value of less than 1pg/ml with reduced plasma osmolality. Urinary vasopressin was also elevated and immunoreactive material was found in the tumour tissue.

Antebi, Malinsky, Sors and Veron (1974) described how investigation of a patient with the Lambert-Eaton Syndrome in conjunction with SIADH led to the discovery of a pulmonary tumour. The patient was 36 years old and was found to have a plasma sodium of 127 m equiv. They subsequently found an undifferentiated tumour in the right lung.

Central Nervous System Disease and Hypothalamic Dysfunction.

Many central nervous lesions have been associated with SIADH. This could be a result either of damage to the hypothalamo-neurohypophysial system or to abnormal stimulation at the hypothalamic nuclei. Munoz, Valencia, Lopez and Junko (1975) have described the syndrome in association with CNS infections. They studied 58 patients with either meningitis, infective polyneuritis or poliomyelitis and one patient with intracranial tumour and detected the syndrome in around 10% of the patients studied. Satisfactory management of the conditions was achieved by restriction of the fluid intake.

During the year Raskind, Orenstein and Christopher (1975) published their observations on three post-menopausal women with psychotic depression. These patients exhibited polydipsia and electrolyte patterns suggestive of inappropriate vasopressin production. Immunoassay was performed on plasma from one of the patients and a concentration of 4.1 μU/ml was found. This was clearly inappropriate for the concurrent plasma sodium which was 117mmol/l, since, with this assay, plasma vasopressin following 14h dehydration in a control subject was found to be 2.3 μU/ml. The increased vasopressin secretion, these authors suggest, reflects the underlying dysfunction of the hypothalamus and limbic system of the brain. They did not feel that it represented non-specific release associated with the altered emotional state.

Thoracic Disease

The mechanism underlying increased ADH production in pulmonary disease is not clear. Ectopic ADH production has been suggested in pulmonary tuberculosis, but is unlikely to be the cause in other disease states. Since atrial receptors have been implicated in ADH release, reduced atrial pressure could be the cause both in intrathoracic disease and during positive pressure ventilation. Hypoxia has also been shown to stimulate vasopressin secretion (Forsling and Ullmann 1974; Alexander, Forsling, Martin, Nixon, Ratcliffe, Redstone and Turnbridge, 1972), so that reduced arterial $p0_2$ could be a contributory factor.

A case of inappropriate secretion of vasopressin in thoracic disease was presented by Spanos and Spry (1974) in the British Medical Journal, which subsequently generated some correspondence in the same journal. They described a patient with a chronic chest infection, a plasma osmolality of 269 mosm/l and a urinary osmolality of 684 mosm/l. They also claim to have found vasopressin in the urine at this time. Unfortunately, no indication is given of the assay method used nor the concentration of AVP. Nevertheless they claimed, rather dogmatically, that on the basis of this finding, there can be no doubt about the diagnosis of SIADH. Admittedly, Miller and Moses (1972) have shown that vasopressin is generally undetectable in the urine with a plasma osmolality of less than 283 mosm/l. This does, however, depend on the assay used. With some antisera positive values could be found in such circumstances. Water restriction and antibiotics were successfully used to treat the patient. As the syndrome was cured with antibiotics, it was suggested that the infective tissue was involved in excess production of vasopressin. The patient was reported to be cyanosed so that hypoxia might also be involved. Myers (1974), on the other hand, suggests that stimulation of the sympathetic afferent fibres or B1 receptor sites could play a part due to pressure changes caused by the inflammatory process. He also takes issue with the treatment used by Spanos and Spry, claiming the fluid restriction may be a hazard because of possible thickening of the bronchial mucosa. Tetracycline too, should be avoided as this is a diuretic and can cause vasopressin release through volume depletion.

The paper by Spanos and Spry also prompted Little and Dowdle (1975) to report to the British Medical Journal inappropriate ADH secretion in a child of 6 with bronchopneumonia due to *Mycoplasma pneumoniae*. The increase in ADH production could be due to any of the factors mentioned above. It is also interesting to speculate whether the observed fever could play a role, since it has been reported that elevated body temperature can provoke vasopressin release (Segar and Moore, 1968; Forsling, Ingram and Stanier, 1975). Mor, Ben-Galim and Abrahamov (1975) also found SIADH associated with pneumonia in an infant. Hyponatraemia in pneumonia is often reported in adults but rarely in children.This could be due to the fact that pneumonia in childhood is easily treated and any associated hyponatraemia would be short-lived and go undetected. Mor et al, also feel that ADH, in cases of pneumonia, is produced by reduction of pressure in the left atrium, resulting from pulmonary vasoconstriction produced by hypoxia. They present a flow diagram linking all the factors involved and attributing the continued naturesis, which is difficult to account for, to release of third factor and inhibition of aldosterone. Although this is a plausible explanation it is highly speculative. Their diagram also indicates that elevated ADH results in increased water ingestion. Whether the authors intended this or not, it is an interesting concept. Fitzsimons (1975) has summarised the evidence for an effect of vasopressin on water intake and this possibility is discussed further in chapter 8.

Schorn (1974) presents further evidence for the incidence of SIADH in pulmonary tuberculosis. He investigated two subjects who adequately fulfilled the criteria for the syndrome. It appears that the syndrome can be found in about 10% of tuberculosis cases.

Another chest condition, in which elevated plasma vasopressin might be found, is in chronic obstructive lung disease. Many patients in this group are unable to excrete a water load normally, although their cardiac function is unimpaired and there is no overt evidence of oedema. White and Woodings (1971) have shown that this defect is more closely related to the elevated pCO_2 than to reduced arterial pO_2 and suggest that it could be due to abnormal renal function. It is possible, however, that since elevated pCO_2 has been shown to stimulate vasopressin release (Philbin, Baratz and Patterson, 1970; Forsling and Rees, 1975) increases in the hormone concentration could contribute to water retention. Farber, Bright, Strawbridge, Robertson and Manfredi (1975) therefore applied the sensitive immunoassay (mentioned above) to the determination of plasma vasopressin concentration after a water load in a group of control subjects and patients with stable non-oedematosis obstructive airway disease. Urinary excretion patterns were also followed. The patients were divided into two groups, those with unaltered and those with elevated pCO_2. These workers could find no evidence that the impaired water excretion was in any way related to altered vasopressin metabolism. The plasma AVP levels were, if anything, lower than normal in the patients and this appeared to be a reflection of the reduced plasma osmolality. Plasma osmolality and vasopressin also fell in the usual way in both groups of patients after the water load. It was confirmed that the impaired water excretion was related to the pCO_2 and to impaired sodium secretion. This suggests that the reduced sodium excretion was due to abnormal blood flow or to increased bicarbonate reabsorption resulting from the hypercapnia.

Drugs

Of the causes of SIADH listed in table I, no reports have appeared this year on the possibility of the syndrome occurring in association with endocrine disorders. Cases have been reported of hyponatraemia associated with drug therapy. De Rivera (1975) noted hyponatraemia in the face of high urinary osmolality in a schizophrenic receiving fluphenazine therapy. In view of the report by Mor and his coworkers, the condition could be related to schizophrenia itself, but de Rivera feels this is unlikely as it was temporally related to the administration of the drug. SIADH following fluphenazine therapy has not been reported previously and the underlying factors are unknown. In general though, there is some controversy as to the mechanism by which drugs produce the syndrome. Basically two hypotheses have been put forward: first that the drugs act to increase the secretion of vasopressin from the neurohypophysis and second that they "sensitise" the kidney to AVP. Direct estimates of plasma AVP (Frahm and Smejkal, 1969; Meinders, Cejka and Robertson, 1974) failed to resolve the problem. In considering such cases, however, one should not forget, as Myers emphasises, the possibility of volume depletion resulting from the diuretic action of the drugs used.

Stuart, Cuaso, Miller and Oski (1975) described a case of recurrent increased secretion of vasopressin following repeated doses of vincristine, a drug used in the treatment of leukaemia. Since hyponatraemia associated with vincristine therapy was first described in 1966, several similar reports have appeared. Robertson, Bhoopalam and Zelkowitz (1973) found elevated vasopressin in 3 patients with this syndrome. The case Stuart et al report was a child receiving treatment for acute lymphatic leukaemia. Symptomatic hyponatraemia was noted 8-10 days after vincristine in association with increased urinary excretion of vasopressin. It could be managed with vigorous fluid restriction. Patients treated with vincristine often show signs of neurotoxicity, so it is possible that alterations in vasopressin release are due to direct neurotoxic effects on the hypothalamo-neurohypophysial system.

Treatment of SIADH

In most of the cases described above relatively normal electrolyte balance was restored by water restriction and conventional therapy of the underlying disease. This form of therapy takes some time to become effective and is therefore inadequate in severe cases. Intravenous administration of hypertonic sodium chloride solution has been tried in this situation. It is not satisfactory in the long term as sodium chloride is rapidly excreted. Frusemide has been administered to these patients (Hantman, Rossier, Zohlman and Schrier, 1973) to promote a diuresis. Fluid replacement is then given in the form of a relatively hypertonic solution. This therapy, however, has the disadvantage that it needs very careful monitoring. Mineralocorticoids produce sodium retention and have been used in therapy (Greenberg and Yudi, 1971), but again the benefit is short-lived. An ideal form of therapy would be an antagonist of vasopressin action. Synthetic analogues of vasopressin, some of which have been shown to block its action, may prove of value in the future, but have not as yet been used in patients. However, another established inhibitor of vasopressin action is lithium (see chapter 17). It has been used by White and Fetner (1975) to treat hyponatraemia in a patient with head injuries. Within hours of the administration of lithium carbonate (300 mg every 8h) a maintained diuresis was seen. Sodium excretion ceased and within two days the urinary osmolality had fallen to 187 mosm/l. and the plasma osmolality was normal. The drug was not continued and thereafter there was a gradual fall in the plasma sodium content. No change in urinary cyclic AMP was found during lithium administration which the authors take to be further evidence that lithium acts at a step beyond the formation of cAMP in response to vasopressin (see chapter 10). They suggest that lithium carbonate may be an effective treatment for SIADH. There are several risks associated with the administration of lithium including possible lithium intoxication. Lithium obviously cannot be used in all situations and in any event should only be used with extreme care and constant clinical and laboratory monitoring.

Landolt (1974) has used diphenylhydantoin successfully in the treatment of inappropriate vasopressin which occurred in an 8 year old after surgery for craniopharyngioma. A dose of 250 mg every 8h was used. The syndrome reversed shortly after the second dose and the serum sodium levels soon returned to normal. When the drug was withdrawn urinary concentration was again seen to be abnormal. Diphenylhydantoin was less effective when given a second time so that fluid was restricted. This drug probably acts by inhibiting release of vasopressin from the pituitary (Guzek, Russell and Thorn, 1974).

Treatment of the underlying condition obviously presents problems which may not be resolved until the mechanisms resulting in the syndrome are identified. In the case of cancer patients it appears that increased hormone secretion is a result of ectopic hormone production. The cause of elevated secretion in central nervous system disease, as in thoracic disease, has yet to be identified conclusively.

Summary and Conclusions

The many reports of SIADH which have appeared during the year show that, in certain areas of clinical practice, it is a syndrome which should be borne in mind. Until recently there were few reports of plasma ADH concentrations in patients with SIADH. Such measurements have now been made and it appears that in cancer the vasopressin concentration is elevated, albeit modestly. Further measurements are obviously needed, especially in cases of central nervous system and thoracic disease. Such studies may throw further light on the underlying causal mechanisms.

Chapter 17

DIABETES INSIPIDUS

"I said it in Hebrew - I said it in Dutch -
I said it in German and Greek;"

There are a number of causes of production of dilute urine with unaltered or marginally affected GFR, including tubular abnormalities or the administration of certain drugs. Large quantities of dilute urine are generally produced as a result of a deficiency of vasopressin in the neurohypophysis (pituitary diabetes insipidus), by renal resistance to vasopressin (nephrogenic diabetes insipidus) or by excessive consumption of water. Water deprivation tests are used to distinguish between diabetes insipidus (DI) and psychogenic polydipsia. The response of the patient may be monitored by measuring urinary osmolality or directly by estimating vasopressin in urine or plasma. Even with these tests the diagnosis is not always easy to establish; Barrter (1973) reviews this and other tests in more detail.

The cause of DI is damage to the neurohypophysial system, resulting from head injury or the growth of a tumour. Occasionally it occurs as a hereditary condition. It may be treated with a nasal spray of Pitressin or, more recently, lysine vasopressin or by injecting long acting Pitressin. As mentioned in chapter 3, DDAVP (1,deamino-8-D-arginine vasopressin) is a valuable new analogue for use in this condition. A number of other drugs including chlorpropamide or clofibrate have been used in treatment, but apparently are not successful in nephrogenic DI.

Pituitary Diabetes Insipidus

Pituitary DI is not very common, but two cases have been described recently. Kjessler and Lundberg (1974) describe a patient with aspermia, who developed sudden thirst and polydipsia. This would suggest a lesion in the hypothalamus of vascular origin, which first affected the area controlling gonadotrophin secretion and subsequently the synthesis and release of vasopressin.

Lever and his colleagues have reported a case of hypopituitarism with DI (Trust, Brown, Chinn, Lever, Morton, Padfield, Robertson, Ireland, Melville and Thomson, 1975). They also put forward a possible explanation for the observation that there is sometimes a spontaneous alteration of polyuria and rise in urinary osmolality. On investigation, the patient was found to have an inoperable pinealoma. They describe the development of the tumour and the associated impairment of physiological function. Initially the patient presented with headaches, thirst and polyuria which could be controlled with thiazide. Later it appeared that the tumour expanded, destroying the thirst centre, as the patient lost thirst sensation and developed severe dehydration and oliguria. Measurements of plasma vasopressin and angiotensin II were made during the period of severe dehydration. They found that the vasopressin levels were low, but the angiotensin II levels were profoundly elevated. These observations support the suggestion that high angiotensin II levels are largely responsible for the observed oliguria.

Excretion of Cyclic AMP in Diabetes Insipidus

Raij, Perheentupa and Harkonen (1974) have looked at DI in children. They studied the urinary excretion of cyclic AMP (cAMP) with a view to distinguishing between pituitary DI and nephrogenic DI. They found the excretion of cAMP was depressed in both groups of patients, but reported an apparent paradox when they looked at the effect of vasopressin on urinary cAMP. They noted, as expected, that there was no effect in children with nephrogenic DI, but surprisingly, that there was a net fall in urinary cAMP in those with pituitary DI. When they came to consider the results in relation to other parameters of renal function, they found that vasopressin produced an increase in the cAMP: creatinine ratio. Vasopressin therefore appeared to affect urinary cAMP excretion in several ways, so that they consider the measurement of urinary cAMP to be misleading in the differential diagnosis of DI.

Treatment of Diabetes Insipidus

It is well established that the sulphonylurea, chlorpropamide, produces an antidiuresis in patients with DI. Clofibrate and carbamazepine have been shown to have a similar action. These drugs are thought to act either by stimulating release of vasopressin from the neurohypophysis or by enhancing the action of the hormone on the kidney. Chlorpropamide has the drawback that it induces hyperinsulinaemia and hypoglycaemia and therefore the antidiuretic action of other drugs has been investigated. Meinders, Cejka and Robertson (1974) were able to confirm the antidiuretic action of carbamazepine in patients with pituitary DI. The antidiuresis was, in essence, similar to that produced by vasopressin. They measured plasma vasopressin in the six patients investigated and found it to be undetectable in all six patients before and during the administration of carbamazepine. In the two control subjects vasopressin concentration actually fell during the administration of the drug. It would not appear then, to act by stimulating release, or altering clearance of vasopressin. The suggestion was made that it enhances the response to vasopressin or has a direct effect itself on the kidney.

Rado (1975) carried out studies on the three antidiuretic agents, chlorpropamide, carbamazepine and clofibrate. He studied seven patients and, as a result of the information he obtained, suggested that these compounds act by producing a permanent enhancement of either synthesis or release of vasopressin.

Since chlorpropamide is an effective agent in the treatment of DI, the action of other sulphonylurea compounds have been investigated. Paradoxically, many of these have been found to have a diuretic action. Rado, Borbely, Szende and Tako (1974) investigated the effect of glibenclamide in healthy control subjects on the antidiuresis produced by lysine vasopressin. They found that glibenclamide partially blocked the antidiuretic response. This was not felt to be a result of direct interference on the response to lysine vasopressin, but rather through inhibition of sodium reabsorption in the distal tubule, unrelated to vasopressin.

These observations were confirmed for the drug glyburide (a sulphonylurea) by Moses, van Gemert and Miller (1974). They studied the response of three normal subjects to oral administration of glyburide. After three days of treatment vasopressin was infused and the response compared with that seen during a control period. Glyburide did not appear to have an effect on the peripheral action of vasopressin in these healthy hydrated subjects. These workers studied the clearance of ^{125}I-labelled vasopressin in rats with hereditary DI treated with this drug. They also studied the effect of an injection of Pitressin tannate after glyburide therapy. Treatment had no effect on the excretion of labelled vasopressin, which suggests that the unchanged excretion of vasopressin in glyburide treated subjects can be taken as an indication of unchanged secretion. An augmentation of the vasopressin-induced antidiuresis following glyburide was observed. Since glyburide does not appear to interact with vasopressin, it probably has a direct action on the kidney, either on the distribution of blood flow or on the tubule.

Moses and his colleagues are not alone in using rats with hereditary DI as a model for this disease. Laycock, Lee and Lewis (1974) have studied the effect of chlorpropamide on water balance in Brattleboro DI rats treated with Pitressin (25 or 50 mU/24h). They were unable to find any effect on the vasopressin response both in these animals or in glucose hydrated heterozygous (non-DI) rats. This discrepancy is hard to explain.

Mohring, Mohring, Schomig, Schomig-Brekner and Haack (1974) have studied potassium and water balance in DI rats. Potassium deficiency has been reported in these rats which could be the result of the high urinary flows. These workers therefore observed the effect of vasopressin to see if it produced potassium retention. They were able to confirm this suggestion; single injections of vasopressin in the range 50-

500 mU produced a dose related potassium retention. Sodium retention was only induced by the higher doses (250 or 500 mU). They were unable to identify the underlying mechanism, but the response did appear to rely on a reduction in urine flow. It is unlikely that this would be of significance in the normal rat. When considering their observations, Mohring and his associates point out that the maintenance dose of vasopressin given to DI animals should be below that which produces sodium retention, namely 250 mU per animal.

Lithium-induced Polyuria

It is now well established that lithium therapy can be associated with polyuria and polydipsia - a diabetes-like condition. This is said to be a common complaint in psychiatric patients given lithium (Forrest, Cohen, Torretti and Epstein, 1971), although there have been few reported cases. In experimental animals and as early as 1950 Radomski, Fuyat, Nelson and Smith described polyuria in dogs given lithium chloride. In many instances the polyuria was resistant to vasopressin, suggesting that it exerts its action largely on the kidney. Evidence obtained from investigations on mammalian kidney preparations (Dousa and Hechter 1970; Beck, Reed and Davis, 1971) and toad bladder (Singer and Franko, 1973) indicates that interference with the vasopressin-sensitive adenyl cyclase is the underlying cause. The response in the rat has been extensively studied and it seems that this animal is very sensitive to lithium, the syndrome occurring regularly in these animals, but less so in the clinical situation. A possible reason for the predominant action on the kidney could be that this organ selectively accumulates lithium ions. Not all the attention has been directed towards the renal response and studies, such as those of Torp-Pederson and Thorn (1973) on isolated rat neurohypophysis, suggest that the defect may be a result of altered neurohypophysial function. Interpretation of the results of some investigations is difficult because they used concentrations well beyond the therapeutic range. Development of the understanding of the effect of lithium on fluid balance has been summarised in a recent publication: *Lithium, Research and Therapy* (Ed Johnson, 1975), which includes reviews by MacNeil and Jenner, Berens and Wolff, Fyro and Sedvall and by Forn.

Lithium and Renal cAMP

Although lithium is known to act on the cAMP system in the kidney, it is not clear which step is influenced. Dousa (1974) therefore investigated the effect of lithium on preparations of enzymes made from human renal medullary tissue. The 600 g sediment of the tissue homogenate was used for studying adenyl cyclase and the 100,000 g supernatant for studying protein kinase and cAMP phosphodiesterase. In the presence of 200 mM sodium chloride or 200 mM urea plus 100 mM sodium chloride, the addition of lithium chloride inhibited the vasopressin stimulation of adenyl cyclase, but had no effect on the basal activity of the enzyme. Lack of action on the basal activity suggests that lithium does not interfere with the catalytic site of the adenyl cyclase complex. The fact that inhibition was seen at all concentrations of vasopressin used and that analogues of vasopressin with different affinities all inhibited the response, suggests that the inhibition is non-competitive. Dousa (1974) suggests that lithium decreases the number of active receptor sites or interferes with the binding capacity of the receptors or the coupling between the receptors and the catalytic subunits of the membrane adenyl cyclase. The suggestion that lithium acts on the formation of cAMP is reinforced by the finding that cAMP phosphodiesterase activity is not affected by lithium. Protein kinase activity was marginally affected. This may also contribute to the diuretic effect of lithium.

Beck and Davis (1975), using medullary slices of rat kidney, found almost opposite results. They again observed that basal cAMP concentration was little affected by lithium alone and that the drug produced a dose related inhibition of vasopressin stimulation of cAMP. They suggest, however, that this is not a result of inhibition of the formation of cAMP. This suggestion was supported by the observation that 10 mM lithium had no measurable effect on vasopressin stimulated adenyl cyclase but did augment the activity of high Km phosphodiesterase (cAMP, 10^{-4}M). These results suggest that lithium can act by increasing the catabolism of cAMP. They do not, however, rule out the involvement of other steps in lithium inhibition.

Jenner and MacNeil (1975) feel that their results are compatible with the hypothesis that lithium acts to inhibit adenyl cyclase. They observed, in chronically lithium-treated rats, that there was an increase in antidiuretic activity in the urine. They feel that this results from the response of the neurohypophysial sysem to the fluid loss caused by lithium.

Lithium and Electrolyte Balance

Hochman and Gutman (1974) have considered the effect of lithium on the neurohypophysis. In order to determine the relationship between lithium-induced responses and vasopressin, they used Brattleboro rats with hereditary DI. They followed the effect of lithium on water and electrolyte balance in control rats, DI rats and DI rats treated with vasopressin. They estimated the vasopressin content of the pituitary in the control rats and, in addition, the effect on the adenyl cyclase activity of cell membrane preparations from the kidney of both control and DI rats. They were able to confirm that lithium has an effect on the vasopressin stored in the neurohypophysis. This effect was not specific for lithium and did not appear to be the principle underlying the mechanism of action of lithium. They observed, as other workers have done, that lithium produced an increased water intake and excretion. Similar effects were seen in DI rats maintained on injections of Pitressin tannate. Since lithium has the same effect on control and DI rats it is unlikely that it alters the production or secretion of vasopressin. Additional evidence came from the observation that lithium has no effect on adenyl cyclase prepared from kidneys of rats with DI.

It seems that lithium may have an effect independent of that on vasopressin. It was able to increase urine volume and water intake in untreated rats with DI. Lithium also produced a fall in potassium excretion although it had no effect on sodium. Hochman and Gutman (1974) therefore suggested that aldosterone may be involved.

Martinez-Maldonado, Stavroulaki-Tsapara, Tsaparas, Suki and Eknoyan (1975) interpret their results as indicating that lithium treatment may result in impaired vasopressin release. They found that, in rats treated with lithium, dibutyryl cAMP and vasopressin could produce a response, albeit reduced. They speculate that impairment of release or a block in the distal part of the kidney is involved. The possibility that chronic administration of lithium was affecting proximal tubular absorption is supported by the observation that while the diluting capacity of the kidney is normal there is increased excretion of phosphate and uric acid. This lends support to a vasopressin-independent action of lithium on the kidney.

Hoeg and Andersen (1975) report a case of lithium-induced DI in a patient with manic depressive psychosis. It was not a permanent condition and could be improved by infusion of vasopressin. The authors suggest, in contrast to much of the work summarised above, that in this case lithium had operated by its influence on central nervous system pathways.

Summary and Conclusions

Most studies which have been performed during the year on diabetes insipidus have been devoted to drugs which may be used to treat the condition, and their mode of action. Those drugs which have been studied are chlorpropamide carbamazepine and clofibrate. There is some disagreement as to the way in which they act; however, the general concensus seems to be that they have a direct action on the kidney rather than affecting secretion of vasopressin. Lithium-induced polyuria has also been the subject of investigation. After lithium treatment the vasopressin-stimulated increase in cyclic AMP is reduced. This could be due to an effect on formation or destruction of the nucleotide.

Chapter 18

ARTERIAL VASOPRESSIN INFUSION

"That's exactly the method, the Bellman
In a hasty parenthesis cried,"

Although vasopressin has a general effect on vascular smooth muscle, certain vessels, as mentioned in chapter 3, are particularly sensitive to the hormone. The splanchnic area represents one such region, and hence the hormone lowers portal venous pressure. This fact obviously renders vasopressin a suitable candidate for use in controlling oesophageal variceal bleeding. Intravenous infusion of vasopressin was first used in the management of variceal haemorrhage by Kehne and his colleagues in 1956. There are, however, dangers in the systemic use of vasopressin. These include a decrease in cardiac output, vasoconstriction of the coronary arteries and water retention, resulting from the antidiuretic effect. Nusbaum, Baum, Sakiyalak and Blakemore in 1967 therefore employed infusions into the superior mesenteric artery, and by this means lower doses could be used, thus reducing the side effects. This form of therapy is, however, still the subject of controversy. Many enthusiastic clinical reports have appeared, but it has been questioned e.g. by Donaldson (1970). In an effort to evaluate the advantages and possible hazards associated with this form of treatment, investigations have been carried out on dogs, with particular interest in the risk of causing liver ischaemia. Although care obviously must be taken in extrapolating results on dogs to patients with cirrhosis, nevertheless valuable additional data have been obtained from animal studies.

Studies on Dogs

Although one serious side effect of vasopressin infusion is a reduction in coronary blood flow and cardiac output, the relative changes in these have not been systematically studied and so Fisher, Sheff, Novak and White (1974) investigated the effect of intra-arterial infusion in 13 dogs. Cardiac output and coronary flow were estimated using electronic flow probes round the ascending aorta and on a segment of the circumflex branch of the left coronary artery. They reported premature ventricular contractions and found that both cardiac output and coronary flow fell to a minimum between 15 and 45 min after the beginning of the infusion. With doses of 0.2 and 0.40 U/min the coronary blood flow fell by 25% and 35% respectively and the cardiac output by 47% and 63%. The reduction in cardiac output was accompanied by a fall in both heart rate and stroke volume. In these studies the doses of vasopressin were comparable with those used in clinical practice (0.1 - 0.4U/min).

The authors do not feel that these results contraindicate the use of intra-arterial vasopressin. However, they do recommend, especially in the case of older individuals, that careful monitoring of the patient's cardiac status be carried out during and after the treatment.

Barr, Lakin and Rosch (1975) also reported a fall in cardiac output following AVP infusions in a study in which they compared the effects of intra-arterial and intravenous infusions. This fall was of the order of 26% following arterial infusion at a rate of 2.75 mU/Kg/min (i.e. approximately 0.055 - 0.0825 U/min or equivalent to 0.2 U/min in man). They also found a 55% fall in blood flow in the superior mesenteric artery and 44% in the portal vein. Portal pressure fell by 25% and systemic blood pressure increased by 27%. These changes were not significantly different from those seen when the same infusion was given intravenously. These findings would suggest that the relatively more easily administered intravenous infusion could be used in the management of bleeding from varices. Clinical studies, including a series in which a catheter was wedged in an hepatic vein or introduced into an umbilical vein, would obviously need to be performed before this technique could be adopted.

Selective infusion into a superior mesenteric artery through an aberrant hepatic artery has not been advised because of possible liver ischaemia. In order to evaluate this possibility Barr, Lakin and Rosch (1975) measured the flow in the hepatic, splenic, left gastric and superior mesenteric arteries in the dog, again using electromagnetic flow meters. Twenty dogs were used in the investigation in which it was found that during vasopressin infusion there was a persistent decrease of flow in all the arteries, save the hepatic artery. A biphasic response was seen in hepatic arterial flow with infusions of 0.1 mU/Kg/min to 8.4 mU/Kg/min. After a sharp drop, the flow rapidly increased to above the initial level, where it remained until the end of the infusion. It is thought that this response was due to autoregulatory dilatation in the liver resulting from a decrease in portal flow. This response with dilatation of the arterioles and small arteries in the liver is favourable evidence for the safety of infusion into the superior mesenteric or coeliac artery. The authors do, however, emphasise that further experimental work is required to evaluate the safety of prolonged arterial infusion, especially in patients with advanced cirrhosis and complete reversal of portal flow. Fingeroth, Storer, Ramsby and Conn (1973) also reported that after the initial reduction there was a secondary increase in blood flow through the liver. Another possible danger of vasopressin infusion is the hypoxia which could result from intra-arterial infusion. Jacobson, Pawlick, Mailman, Burks and Shepherd (1974) therefore investigated the effect of vasoconstrictors on intestinal oxygen consumption. They looked at the effect of vasopressin, in doses of 0.3 and 0.7 mU/Kg/min, angiotensin II, prostaglandin F_{2a} and adrenaline (after β blockade). They found that the higher dose of vasopressin produced a 22% fall in oxygen consumption and even the lower dose, which had no effect on blood flow, resulted in a drop in oxygen consumption by 6%. Adrenaline alone had no effect on oxygen consumption.

In the present context another clinical application of vasopressin could be the control of post-hepatectomy portal hypertension and splanchnic sequestration of blood. This often complicates major hepatic resection. Sirinek and Thomford (1973) found that in dogs, post-operative administration of vasopressin minimised the increase in portal pressure associated with major hepatic resection. Administration of isoprenaline to reduce the vasopressin-induced fall in cardiac output was also successful.

Clinical Studies

Although these studies in the dog seem to indicate that vasopressin infusions are relatively safe and may be useful in reducing portal hypertension, the clinical evidence is not so clear cut. The possibility, already raised by Barr et al (1975), that there could be a return to venous infusions has been taken up by Thomford and Sirinek. This route of administration is quicker and simpler clinically. In their studies, Thomford and Sirinek (1975) compared the effect of a continuous intravenous infusion with bolus administration in seven patients. Catheters were inserted into the portal vein via the umbilical vein, the superior vena cava and the radial artery to allow continuous monitoring of pressures and cardiac output. Vasopressin was given as a bolus of 15 units in 5 min. or as an infusion of 40 units over 15 min. Both types of treatment produced a similar initial fall in portal venous pressure, but the continuous infusion gave rise to less pronounced generalised cardiovascular and gastrointestinal side effects. Furthermore, as would be expected,the continuous infusion has a more prolonged effect on portal venous pressure.

Most of these reports have come from the United States, but recently reports have appeared from Europe. Aronsen, Wetterlin, Emas, Vojtise, Mulder and Cort (1975) have used the long acting analogue, triglycyl-lysine vasopressin in the treatment of gastrointestinal bleeding (see chapter 3). Amman, Scholl and Vogt (1974) and Markoff, Hobl, Horder, Flury and Ratti (1973) both describe the use of intra-arterial administration of vasopressin. The latter concluded that arterial infusion could help stop the bleeding and allow further time for treatment to be organised. This was also the conclusion of Conn, Ramsby and Storer (1974,1975) who performed a prospective clinical trial comparing vasopressin infusion with conventional treatment such as balloon tamponade or ice water lavage in 60 episodes of upper GI tract haemorrhage. Thirty two patients were treated conventionally and twenty eight were additionally given vasopressin therapy. Surprisingly, survival was not improved in those patients receiving vasopressin despite the fact that bleeding was most effectively controlled from both varices and non-variceal lesions. The chance of survival, even with cessation of haemorrhage, was thought to depend on the degree of advancement of the underlying disease. The massive extent of the haemorrhage and the frequent recurrence could also be important, especially as in some cases vasopressin was given when alternative treatment failed. Vasopressin produced some cardiovascular side-effects in these patients, but probably not sufficient to account for the mortality in this group. Complications such as bacteraemia, thrombosis and embolism are associated with the catheterisation but again there was no evidence that any deleterious side-effects of this nature were involved.

Amidst these fairly optimistic reports on the use of vasopressin infusion Millette, Huet, Lavoie and Viallet (1975) introduce yet another note of caution. During the course of vasopressin infusions of 0.2 U/h they found that they could only produce relatively small decreases (9.6%) in portal venous pressure, smaller than Barr et al found in dogs or Thomford and Sirinek found using a dose of 0.036 U/h intravenously. It should be noted, however, that the dose used in the dog was relatively greater. It would seem, nevertheless, that there is considerable variation in the response of patients to vasopressin. Another explanation could be that all the hormone is not taken up by the liver and passes into the systemic circulation. That this does in fact occur, can be seen from the observation that there was an inverse relationship between the fall in portal venous pressure and cardiac output (which may be taken to reflect systemic concentration of vasopressin). Fairly high levels of vasopressin in the region of 50-100 times physiological levels have been reported in patients undergoing selective arterial mesenteric infusion (Baum, Coggins, Misch and Athanasoulis, 1974), the estimates being made by radioimmunoassay. Despite these high levels the authors say that there were no adverse effects on renal function. Nusbaum and Conn (1975) in their editorial "Science or Sceance" take up this report of Millette and his colleagues and discuss the differences between their observations and those of other workers. They compared their own data with that of Millette and other workers and did show that 85% of non-bleeding patients show a decrease in portal pressure with vasopressin infusion into the superior mesenteric artery, whereas only 43% showed a decrease during variceal bleeding. Amongst other explanations they considered the remote possibility that the vasopressin exerted its beneficial effect by contraction of the smooth muscle of the oesophagus, which could then compress the varices.

Another consistent effect produced by vasopressin in the studies of Millette et al was a reduction in the arterial pO_2 from a mean of 77.3 to 66.9 mmHg and a fall in the portal pO_2 from 47.8 to 38.8 mmHg, which would suggest reduced blood flow through the splanchnic tissues. A decrease in pO_2 following AVP infusion in man has not previously been reported. However, in no other studies was the initial pO_2 as low as in this investigation. Decreased portal pO_2 must of course be taken into account when this approach is used in cirrhotic patients.

The discussion so far has largely centered on treatment of lesions in the upper GI tract - bleeding from oesophageal varices or secondary to portal hypertension, but intra-arterial infusion has been used in patients with upper and lower GI tract haemorrhage. Geronilla, Sampliner and Lerner (1975) report early successes with infusions into the coeliac or superior mesenteric artery of patients with GI bleeding from a number of different causes in a number of different areas. The initial selective infusion stopped the haemorrhage in 13 patients (76.5%), but in 4 of the patients there was subsequent bleeding. Variceal and non-variceal bleeds were controlled equally successfully. Encouraged by this success they feel that more extensive clinical trials should be performed.

Athanasoulis, Baum, Rosch, Waltman, Ring, Smith, Sugarbuter and Wood (1975) are equally enthusiastic about the use of arterial infusions of vasopressin to arrest bleeding from colonic diverticulosis. They have extended an earlier study (Baum, Rosch, Dotter, Ring, Athanasoulis, Waltman and Courey, 1973) in order to investigate the longer term progress of the patients. As a result of their study on 24 patients, they feel that once the intravascular volume has been replaced, mesenteric angiography should be performed which not only localises the site of bleeding, but allows the infusion of vasopressin. In their investigation they claim that the hormone controlled bleeding in 22 of the 24 cases. Vasopressin infusions alone may not prevent bleeding but can obviate the need for emergency surgery under adverse conditions. Segmental colectomy can be performed once the site of the lesion has been identified angiographically and this seems to be as effective as subtotal colectomy in preventing recurrent bleeding.

A paper has also appeared during the year which describes the treatment of small intestinal haemorrhage with vasopressin infusion. Although uncommon in Western Europe and the United States, cases of typhoid fever still occur, the two major accompanying complications being haemorrhage and intestinal perforation. Recurrent haemorrhage in these cases may be treated by surgical removal of the section of the small intestine involved, but as with most emergency surgery of the GI tract the mortality rate is high. Collins, Ball and Dorsey (1975) therefore tried using the vasopressin infusion. The hormone was administered at rates of 0.2 - 0.4 units per minute through an angiographic catheter located near the origin of the ileocolic branch of the superior mesenteric artery. After 6h of infusion at the higher rate the bleeding stopped completely. The abrupt cessation of bleeding which accompanied vasopressin infusion led the authors to believe that it was due to the action of vasopressin and did not occur spontaneously.

In most of the studies on cirrhotic patients the effects of vasopressin administration alone was studied. Sirinek and Thomford (1975a,b) however, have looked at the effect of added isoprenaline. It was hoped that this addition would prevent the reduction in cardiac output produced by the vasopressin. They found, as did Millette et al, that the changes in cardiac output during vasopressin infusion were variable, but in those patients who did experience a vasopressin-induced fall in cardiac output, isoprenaline was able to suppress the response. It did not appear to affect the reduction in portal venous pressure. This observation may well be of value in clinical practice. A potential benefit of adding isoprenaline could be the reported increase in coronary blood flow (Dedichen and Schenk, 1970).

Prevention of Vasopressin-induced Gastric Erosions

Apart from the adverse cardiovascular effects, systemic infusions of vasopressin have been shown to produce gastric erosions. Dutton, Chin and Hinchey (1975) have examined the erosive potential of intra-arterial vasopressin infusion on the gastric mucosa of pigs. The three hour infusion, given at a rate of 0.2 units per minute, resulted in mucosal damage which resembled clinical and experimental stress erosions. This was prevented by the gastric instillation of a cholestyramine glucose solution. Such findings may be of value in the management of patients receiving arterial vasopressin for upper GI tract bleeding.

Radioprotective Effects of Vasopressin

A hazard accompanying the use of radiotherapy for treatment of tumours in the abdominal and splanchnic region is the damaging effect of ionising radiation on the gastro-intestinal tract and liver. Gray, Conger, Ebert, Hornsey and Scott (1953) described a decrease in the radiosensitivity of tissues whose oxygen tension is reduced. The radioprotective effects of local infusions of vasoconstrictor agents have therefore been investigated. Casarella, Gerstein, Chang, Wolf and Harisiades (1974) have examined the protective effect on the small intestine of infusion of 0.4 U/min vasopressin into mongrel dogs. They found that whereas doses of 1500 rad to control animals were fatal, those animals receiving vasopressin infusions could tolerate a single dose of 2500 rad. In chronic experiments doses of 6000 rad given over six weeks were tolerated. It would appear on the basis of these experiments that the deleterious effects of radiation therapy on the small bowel can be reduced by selective infusion of vasopressin.

Rappleye, Johnson, Olsen and Lagasse (1975) also report favourably on the effect of vasopressin on the response of the gastro-intestinal tract to irradiation. They assessed the radiation protective effect of vasopressin in 300 mice. Median lethal doses were determined for control and vasopressin-treated animals subjected to radiation over the whole abdomen. There was a significant difference in the tolerance of control and vasopressin-treated animals, the latter group withstanding higher doses.

Summary and Conclusions

The therapeutic use of vasopressin has progressed far since Rist described the use of pituitrin in the treatment of bleeding in 1913. However, it appears that there is still a great deal to be learnt about the use of intra-arterial infusions of vasopressin in preventing bleeding from the GI tract. Disagreement about the value of this form of therapy persists. Most authors, however, agree that the technique is valuable in stopping bleeding thereby buying time, so that surgery can be carried out on a semi-elective basis.

REFERENCES

The titles of papers published in languages other than English, Spanish, French, German and Danish have been translated into English.

Abramow M, Dratwa M. Studies with cytochalasin B in the isolated rabbit collecting tubule. Possible role of microfilaments in vasopressin action. In *INSERM* colloquium, p 133, Physiologie du Nephron, Mecanismes et Regulation, 1974a.

Abramow M, Dratwa M. Interaction of vasopressin and diuretics on the isolated rabbit collecting tubule. Eur J Clin Invest 14, 353, 1974b.

Abramow M, Dratwa M. Effect of vasopressin on the isolated human collecting duct. Nature 250, 492-493, 1974c.

Acher R. Chemistry of the neurohypophysial hormones: an example of molecular evolution. In *Handbook of Physiology*, pp 119-130, Section 7, Endocrinology Volume IV. The pituitary gland and its neuroendocrine control, part 1, eds. RO Greep, EB Astwood. American Physiological Society, Washington, 1974.

Acher R, Chauvet J. La structure de la vasopressine de boeuf. Biochim Biophys Acta 12, 487-488, 1953.

Acher R, Fromageot P. The relationship of oxytocin and vasopressin to active proteins of posterior pituitary origin. in *The Neurohypophysis,* pp 39-50, ed. H Heller, Butterworths, London, 1957.

Alexander DP, Bashore RA, Britton HG, Forsling ML. Maternal and foetal arginine-vasopressin in the chronically catheterised sheep. Biol Neonate 25, 242-248, 1974.

Alexander DP, Britton HG, Forsling ML. Oxytocin and antidiuretic hormone release and turnover in the sheep foetus, lamb and ewe. Biol Neonate (in press) 1976.

Alexander DP, Britton HG, Forsling ML, Nixon DA, Ratcliffe JG. The concentrations of adrenocorticotrophin, vasopressin and oxytocin in the foetal and maternal plasma of sheep in the latter half of gestation. J Endocrinol 49, 179-180, 1971.

Alexander DP, Britton HG, Forsling ML, Nixon DA, Ratcliffe JG. Adrenocorticotrophin in foetal sheep and the response to stress. In *The Endocrinology of Pregnancy and Parturition. Experimental Studies in the Sheep*. pp 112-125, ed. CG Pierrepoint, Alpha Omega Alpha Publishing, Cardiff, 1973.

Alexander DP, Britton HG, Forsling ML, Nixon DA, Ratcliffe JG. Pituitary and plasma concentrations of adrenocorticotrophin, growth hormone, vasopressin and oxytocin in foetal and maternal sheep during the latter half of gestation and the response to haemorrhage. Biol Neonate 24, 206-219, 1974.

Alexander DP, Forsling ML, Martin MJ, Nixon DA, Ratcliffe JG, Redstone D, Turnbridge D. The effect of maternal hypoxia on foetal hormone release in the sheep. Biol Neonate 21, 219-229, 1972.

Al-Merani SAMA, Chapman BJ, Munday KA. The sodium ion retaining action of antiotensin II in the rat; inhibition of this action by vasopressin. in *INSERM Colloquium,* p 137, Physiologie du Nephron, Mecanismes et Regulation, 1974.

Altura BM. Neurohypophyseal hormones and analogues: rat pressor potency versus contractile potency on rat arterioles and arteries. Proc Soc Exp Biol Med 146, 1054-1060, 1974.

Altura BM. Magnesium-neurohypophyseal hormone interactions in contraction of vascular smooth muscle. Am J Physiol 228, 1615-1620, 1975a.

Altura BM. Neurohypophyseal hormones and analogues: magnesium dependence and contraction of arterial smooth muscle. Proc Soc Exp Biol Med 148, 1031-1037, 1975b.

Altura BM. Dose-response relationships for arginine vasopressin and synthetic analogs on three types of rat blood vessels: possible evidence for regional differences in mammalian receptor sites within a mammal. J Pharmacol Exp Ther 193, 413-423, 1975.

Altura BM. Sex and estrogens and responsiveness of terminal arterioles to neurohypophyseal hormones and catecholamines. J Pharmacol Exp Ther 193, 403-412, 1975c.

Altura BM, Altura BT, Hershey SG. Pharmacodynamic actions of corticosteroids on the microcirculation and vascular smooth muscle. in *Steroids and Shock.* pp 67-87, ed. TM Glenn, University Park Press, Baltimore, 1974.

Altura BM, Malaviya D, Reich CF, Orkin LR. Effects of vaso-active agents on isolated human umbilical arteries and veins. Am J Physiol 222, 345-353, 1972.

Amman J, Scharli H, Vogt B. Die selektive intrarterielle Vasopressin infusion bei Behandlung von Blutungen des obern Gastrointestinaltraks. Helv Chir Acta 41, 147-150, 1974.

Anderson RJ, Cadnapaphornchai P, Harbottle JA, McDonald KM, Schrier RW. Mechanism of effect of thoracic inferior vena cava constriction on renal water excretion. J Clin Invest 54, 1473-1479, 1974.

Anderson RJ, Berl T, McDonald KM, Schrier RW. Evidence for an in vivo antagonism between vasopressin and prostaglandin in the mammalian kidney. J Clin Invest 56, 420-426, 1975.

Andersson B. The central control of water and salt balance. In *Neural Integration of Physiological Mechanisms.* pp 213-225, eds. CL Mogenson, FR Calaresu, University of Toronto Press, 1975.

Andrews P. Estimation of molecular weights of proteins by Sephadex gel-filtration. Biochem J 91, 222-233, 1964.

Aronson AS, Svenningsen NW. DDAVP test for estimation of renal concentrating capacity in infants and children. Arch Dis Child 49, 654-659, 1974.

Antebi L, Malinsky M, Sors C, Veron M. Syndrome de Lambert-Eaton et Syndrome de Schwartz-Barrter: un cas d'association revelateur d'un cancer pulmonaire. Narve Presse Med 3, 2169-2172, 1974.

Argy WP, Handler JS, Orloff JS. Ca^{++} and Mg^{++} effects on toad bladder response to cyclic AMP, theophylline and ADH analogs. Am J Physiol 213, 803-808, 1967.

Aronsen KF, Wetterling S, Emas S, Vojtise KV, Mulder JL, Cort JH. Die Wirkung von Triglycyl-lysin-vasopressin auf Kontrollpersonen und Patienten mit Blutungen des oberen Gastrointestinaltraktes. Klin Wschenschr 53, 747-753, 1975.

Athanasoulis CA, Baum S, Rosch MD, Waltman AC, Ring EJ, Smith JC, Sugarbuter E, Wood W. Mesenteric arterial infusions of vasopressin for haemorrhage from colonic diverticulosis. Am J Surg 129, 212-216, 1975.

Axman G, Fulgraff G. Effects of furosemide on sodium content and transport pool in frog skin. Naunyn Schmiedebergs Arch Pharmacol 290, 275-282, 1975.

Bailey DJ, France VM, Parry HM, Stanier MW. Mammalian foetal skin and urinary bladder: a model for distal nephron function. in Proceeding of Vth Int. Conf. Nephrology, C69, Florence, 1975.

Bakker HR, Dyball REJ. Reduced depletion of neurohypophysial hormone stores by vasopressin administration in rats drinking 2% sodium chloride. Neuroendocrinology 18, 92-103, 1975.

Bakker HR, Dyball REJ, Jones CW. The neurohypophysial content of vasopressin oxytocin and neurophysins A, B and C in rats injected with pitressin tannate. J Endocrinol 65, 60P, 1975.

Bakker HR, Dyball REJ, Jones CW. Increased neural lobe content of neurophysins in rats treated with exogenous vasopressin. Nature 225, 734-735, 1975.

Bar HP, Hechter O, Schwartz IL, Walter R. Neurohypophyseal hormone-sensitive adenyl cyclase of toad urinary bladder. Proc Natl Acad Sci USA 67, 7-12,1970.

Bargmann W. Uber die neurosekretorische Verknupfung von Hypothalamus und Neurohypophyse. Z. Zellforsch Mikroskop Anat 34, 610-634, 1949.

Barker JL, Crayton JW, Nicoll RA. Antidromic and orthodromic responses of paraventricular and supraoptic neurosecretory cells. Brain Res 33, 353-366, 1971.

Barker JL, Ifshin MS, Gainer H. Studies on bursting pacemaker potential activity in molluscan neurons: III. Effects of hormones. Brain Res 84, 501-513, 1975.

Barnes LD, Dousa TP. Effects of adenine nucleotides on the in vitro polymerisation of tubulin from bovine renal medulla. Adv Cyclic Nucleotide Res 5, 831, 1975.

Barnes LD, Engel AG, Dousa TP. Studies on in vitro polymerisation of tubulin from renal medullary extracts. Biochim Biophys Acta 405, 422-433, 1975.

Barnes LD, Hui YSF, Dousa TP. Interaction of ethacrynic acid and cysteine with renal medullary adenylate cyclase. Life Sci 16, 255-262, 1975.

Barnes LD, Hui YSF, Frohnert PP, Dousa TP. Subcellular distribution of the enzymes related to the cellular action of vasopressin on renal medulla. Endocrinology 96, 119-128, 1975.

Barr JW, Lakin RC, Rosch J. Vasopressin and hepatic artery. Effect of selective coeliac infusion of vasopressin on the hepatic artery flow. Invest. Radiol 10, 200-205, 1975.

Barr JW, Lakin RC, Rosch J. Similarity of arterial and intravenous vasopressin on portal and systemic hemodynamics. Gastroenterology 69, 13-19,1975.

Barrter FC. Vasopressin. 5. Clinical evaluation of hormone excess and deficiency. Methods Invest Diagn Endocrinol 2A, 672-679, 1973.

Barrter FC, Schwartz WB. The syndrome of inappropriate secretion of antidiuretic hormone. Am J Med 42, 790-806, 1967.

Barth T, Le Bars NC, Roy C, Jard S. Hydro-osmotic activity of "carba" analogues of oxytocin and (8-arginine) vasopressin on frog (*Rana Esculanta)* bladder. Eur J Pharmacol 32, 214-220, 1975.

Barth T, Rajerison MR, Roy C, Jard S. Activation of rat kidney adenylate cyclase by vasopressin analogues: lack of correlation with antidiuretic activity. Mol Cell Endocrinol 2, 81-90, 1975.

Barth T, Roy C, Rajerison MR, Jard S. Renal adenylate cyclase activation by amino acylated vasopressin and oxytocin. Mol Cell Endocrinol 2, 69-79, 1975.

Bartsokas SK, Polychronopoulou-Trichopolou A, Kouvelas ED, Charissiadou A, Valsamakis S, Kalaitzidou C. Antidiuretic hormone and lipolysis. Endokrinologie 64, 201-204, 1975.

Baum S, Athanasoulis CA, Waltman AC, Ring EJ. Gastrointestinal hemorrhage. Part II Angiographic diagnosis and control. Adv Surg 7, 149, 1973.

Baum S, Coggins C, Misch AB, Athanasoulis CA. Vasopressin blood levels in patients undergoing selective mesenteric infusion for control of gastrointestinal bleeding. Invest Radiol 9, 327-328, 1974.

Baum S, Rosch J, Dotter CT, Ring EJ, Athanasoulis CA, Waltman AC, Cowrey WR. Selective mesenteric arterial infusions in the management of massive diverticular haemorrhage. New Engl J Med 288, 1269-1272, 1973.

Beardwell CG. Radioimmunoassay of arginine vasopressin in human plasma. J Clin Endocrinol Metab 33, 254-260, 1971.

Beart PM, Kelly JS, Schon F. α-aminobutyric acid in the rat peripheral nervous system, pineal and posterior pituitary. Biochem Soc Trans 2, 266-268, 1974.

Beck N, Davis BB. Effects of lithium on vasopressin-dependent cyclic AMP in rat renal medulla. Endocrinology 97, 202-207, 1975.

Beck N, Kim HP. Effect of acute metabolic acidosis on vasopressin-dependent cyclic AMP in rat kidney. Endocrinology 96, 1552-1558, 1975.

Beck N, Reed SW, Davis BB. Effects of lithium (Li) on renal concentration of cyclic AMP (c AMP). Clin Res Proc 19, 684, 1971.

Beck N, Reed SW, Davis BB. Urinary concentrating defect and vasopressin cyclic

AMP in potassium depletion. In *Proc Vth Int Conf Nephrology,* C55, Florence, 1975.

Beck N, Singh H, Reed HV, Murdaugh HV, Davis BB. Pathogenic role of cyclic AMP in the impairment of renal concentrating ability in acute hypercalcemia. J Clin Invest 54, 1049-1055, 1974.

Bell NH. Evidence for a separate adenylate cyclase system responsive to beta-adrenergic stimulation in the renal cortex of the rat. Acta Endocrinol Kbh 77, 604-611, 1974.

Bennet GW, Edwardson JA. Release of corticotrophin releasing factor and hypophysiotropic substances from isolated nerve endings (synaptosomes). J Endocrinol 65, 33-44, 1975.

Berde B, Boissonnas RA. Basic pharmacological properties of synthetic analogues and homologues of neurohypophysial hormones. In *Handbook of Experimental Pharmacology.* pp 802-870, Vol 23, Neurohypophysial and Similar Polypeptides, Springer Verlag, Berlin, 1968.

Berens SC, Wolff J. The effects of lithium on antidiuretic hormone. In *Lithium Research and Therapy.* pp 465-468, ed. FN Johnson, Academic Press, New York, 1975.

Berl T, Harbottle JA, Schrier RW. Effect of alpha-and beta-adrenergic stimulation on renal water excretion in man. Kidney Int 6, 247-253, 1974.

Berl T, Horowitz J, Czaczkes JW, Wald H, Kleeman CR. Effect of indomethacin (indo) on the action of vasopressin (ADH): evidence for a role of prostaglandins (PG) in the control of renal water excretion in humans and rats. In *Proc Vth Int Conf Nephrology,* C230, Florence, 1975.

Bisset GW, Clark BJ, Haldar J, Harris MC, Lewis GP, Rocha e Silva M. The assay of milk ejecting activity in the rat. Br J Pharmacol 31, 537-549, 1967.

Boesby S, Pedersen SA. The effect of vasopressin in resting gastro-oesophageal sphincter pressure in man. Scan J Gastroenterol 9, 587-590, 1974.

Bohus B, Ader R, De Wied D. Effects of vasopressin on active and passive avoidance behaviour. Horm Behav 3, 191-197, 1972.

Borner E. Untersuchungen uber die klinische Bedeutung des antidiuretischen Hormons. Ann Univ Sarav Med 21, 1-53, 1974.

Borth J, Hutter HJ, Pliska V, Sorm F. Inactivation of deamino oxytocin and deamino-carbo-oxytocin, (D-lys^{8}) - and (D-arg^{8}) vasopressin by kidney cell particles. Experientia 25, 646-647, 1969.

Breslow E. The neurophysins. Adv Enzymol 40, 271-333, 1975a.

Breslow E. On the mechanism of binding of neurohypophyseal hormones and analogs to neurophysins. Ann NY Acad Sci 248, 432-441, 1975b.

Bridges TE, Hillhouse EW, Jones MT. The effect of dopamine on neurohypophysial hormone release in vitro and in vivo. J Physiol Lond 246, 107P-109P, 1975.

Burford GD, Dyball REJ, Moss RL, Pickering BT. Synthesis of both neurohypophysial hormones in both the paraventricular and supraoptic nuclei of the rat. J Anat 117, 261-269, 1974.

Burguburu AM, Geelen G. Determination de la demi-vie de l'hormone antidiuretique (lysine-vasopressine) chez l'homme par methode radioimmunologique. C R Soc Biol Paris 168, 965-970, 1974.

Burlet A, Marchetti J, Duheille J. Immuno-histochemistry of vasopressin: study of the hypothalamo-hypophysial system of normal, dehydrated and hypophysectomized rats. In *Neurosecretion: the Final Common Pathway.* pp 24-30, ed F Knowles, L Vollrath, Springer Verlag, New York, Berlin, 1974.

Burton AM, Forsling ML. Hormone content of the neurohypophysis in foetal newborn and adult guinea pigs. J Physiol Lond 221, 6-7P, 1972.

Cadnapaphornchai P, Boykin JL, Berl T, McDonald KM, Schrier RW. Mechanism of effect of nicotine on renal water excretion. Am J Physiol 227, 1216-1220, 1974.

Carroll L. *The Hunting of the Snark: an Agony in Eight Fits.* McMillan & Co, London, 1876.

Casarella WJ, Gerstein H, Chang C, Wolf MA, Harisiades L. Selective transcatheter pharmacologic protection of the small bowel and liver during radiotherapy. Invest Radiol 9, 321, 1974.

Cash JD, Gader AMA, de Costa J. The release of plasminogen activator and factor 103 to lysine vasopressin, arginine vasopressin, 1-desamino-8-*a*-arginine vasopressin, angiotensin and oxytocin in man. Br J Haematol 27, 363-364, 1974.

Celis ME, Taleisnik S, Walter R. Release of pituitary melanocyte-stimulating hormone by the oxytocin fragment, H Cys-Tyr-ile-Asn-OH. Biochem Biophys Res Commun 54, 564-569, 1971.

Chaiken IM, Randolph RE, Taylor HC. Conformational effects associated with the interaction of polypeptide ligands with neurophysins. Ann NY Acad Sci 248, 442-451, 1975.

Chard T. Posterior pituitary gland. Clin Endocrinol Oxf 4, 89-106, 1975.

Chard T, Hudson CN, Edwards CRW, Boyd NRH. The release of oxytocin and vasopressin by the human fetus during labour. Nature 234, 352-354, 1971.

Civan MM, DiBona DR. Pathways for the movement of ions and water across toad urinary bladder. II Site and mode of action of vasopressin. J Membr Biol 19, 195-220, 1974.

Cohen P, Camier M, Wolff J, Alazard R, Cohen JS, Griffin JH. Studies of bovine neurophysin-neurohypophysial hormone interactions. Ann NY Acad Sci 248, 463-479, 1975.

Cole DF, Nagasubramanian S. Substances affecting active transport across ciliary epithelium and their possible role in determining intraocular pressure. Exp Eye Res 16, 251-264, 1973.

Collins WJ, Ball RE, Dorsey TJ. Typhoid ileitis with hemorrhage. A case report with new therapy. Am J Digest Dis 20, 94-96, 1975.

Conn HO, Ramsby GR, Storer EH. Selective intra-arterial vasopressin in the treatment of upper gastrointestinal hemorrhage. A controlled clinical trial. Gastroenterology 66, A226/880, 1974.

Conn HO, Ramsby GR, Storer EH, Mutchnick P, Joshi H, Phillips MM, Cohen SA, Fields GN, Petroski D. Intra-arterial vasopressin in the treatment of upper gastrointestinal hemorrhage: a prospective controlled clinical trial. Gastroenterology 68, 211-221, 1975.

Cort JH, Albrecht I, Novakova J, Mulder JL, Jost K. Regional and systemic effects of some vasopressins: structural features of the hormone which prolong activity. Eur J Clin Invest 5, 165-175, 1975.

Cort JH, Sedlakova E, Kluh I, Mulder JL. Neurophysin binding and natriuretic peptides from the posterior pituitary. Ann NY Acad Sci 248, 336-344, 1975.

Cort JH, Skopkova J, Schuck O, Stribrna J, Sawyer WH. Indirect characterisation of the antidiuretic receptor (ADR) in the kidneys of man and rat. Eur J Clin Invest 14, 387, 1974.

Cort JH, Skopkova J, Schuck O, Stribrna J, Sawyer WH. Indirect characterisation of the antidiuretic receptor (ADR) in the kidneys of man and rat. In *INSERM Colloquium*, Physiologie du Nephron, p 150, Mecanismes et Regulation 1974.

Cross BA. Functional identification of hypothalamic neurones. In *Recent Studies of Hypothalamic Function.* pp 39-49. Int Symp Calgary, Karger, Basel, 1974.

Cross BA, Dyball REJ. Central pathways for neurohypophysial hormone release. In *Handbook of Physiology,* pp 269-286, Section 7 Endocrinology, Vol 4. The Pituitary Gland and its Neuroendocrine Control Part 1, ed RO Greep, EB Astwood. Amer. Physiological Society, Washington, 1974.

Cuthbert AW, Shum WK. Effects of vasopressin and aldosterone on amiloride binding in toad bladder epithelial cells. Proc R Soc Lond Biol 189, 543-576, 1975.

Cuthbert AW, Wong PYD. Calcium release in relation to permeability changes in toad bladder epithelium following antidiuretic hormone. J Physiol Lond 241, 407-422, 1974.

Cutnell JD, Glasel JA, Hruby VJ. Studies of bovine neurophysin-neurohypophyseal hormone interactions. Ann NY Acad Sci 248, 451-457, 1975.

Darke AC. Studies on the mechanism of potentiation in arteriolar constriction by dexamethasone in vivo. Microvasc Res 9, 317-323, 1975.

Davies R, Forsling ML. Vasopressin release after postural changes and syncope. J Endocrinol 65, 59P-60P, 1975.

Davis BN, Withrington PG. The response of the isolated blood perfused spleen of the dog to angiotensin, oxytocin and vasopressin. Br J Pharmacol 54, 205-212, 1975.

Davis WL, Goodman DBP, Martin JH, Matthews JL, Rasmussen H. Vasopressin induces changes in the toad urinary bladder epithelial surface. J Cell Biol 61, 544-547, 1974.

Davis WL, Goodman DBP, Schuster RJ, Rasmussen H, Martin JH. Effects of cytochalasin B on the response of toad urinary bladder to vasopressin. J Cell Biol 63, 986-997, 1974.

DeBelleroche JA, Bradford HF. The release of endogenous 3,4 dihydroxyphenylethylamine from synaptosomes isolated from corpus striatum. Biochem Soc Trans 3, (1), 99-101, 1975.

DeBodo RC. The antidiuretic activity of morphine and its mechanism. J Pharmacol Exp Therap 82, 74-85, 1944.

Dedichen H, Schenk WG. Haemodynamic effects of isoproterenol and noradrenalin in experimental shock. Acta Chir Scand 139, 213-218, 1973.

Dempsey GP, Bullivant S, Watkins WB. In *Neurosecretion, The Final Neuroendocrine Pathway.* p 301, VI International Symposium, eds F Knowles, L Vollrath, Springer Verlag, New York, 1974.

De Rivera JLG. Inappropriate secretion of antidiuretic hormone from fluphenazine therapy. Ann Intern Med 82, 811-812, 1975.

De Sousa RC, Grosso A, Rufener C. Blockade of hydro-osmotic effect of vasopressin by cytochalasin B. Experientia 30, 175-177, 1974.

De Vitry F, Camier M, Czernichow P, Benda PH, Cohen P, Tixier-Vidal A. Establishment of a clone of mouse hypothalamic neurosecretory cells synthesising neurophysin and vasopressin. Proc Natl Acad Sci USA 71, 3575-3579, 1974.

De Vitry F, Camier M, Czernichow P, Benda P, Cohen P, Tixier-Vidal A. Characterisation of a clonal strain of mouse hypothalamic cells synthesizing neurophysins and vasopressin. Ann NY Acad Sci 248, 64-79, 1975.

De Wied D. The influence of the posterior and intermediate lobe of the pituitary and pituitary peptides on the maintenance of a conditioned avoidance response in rats. Int J Neuropharmacol 4, 157-167, 1965.

De Wied D. The role of the posterior pituitary and its peptides on the maintenance of conditioned avoidance behaviour. *Hormones and Brain Function.* pp 391-397, Budapest 1971, Plenum Press, New York, 1973.

De Wied D, Bohus B, Wimersma Greidanus TJB van. The hypothalamo-neurohypophyseal system and the preservation of conditioned avoidance behaviour in rats. Prog Brain Res 41, 417-428, 1974.

De Wied D, Bohus B, Wimersma Greidanus TJB van. Memory deficit in rats with hereditary diabetes insipidus. Brain Res 85, 152-156, 1975.

Donaldson RM. "Turned off" bleeders. Gastroenterology 59, 477-478, 1970.

Douglas WW. The calcium influx hypothesis and the exocytosis-vesiculation sequence. An interpretation of the mode of secretion of neurohypophysial hormones and significance of microvesicles ('synaptic' vesicles). In *Neurosecretion, the Final Neuroendocrine Pathway.* p 302, VI International Symposium, eds F Knowles, L Vollrath, Springer Verlag, New York, 1974.

Douglas WW. Mechanism of release of neurohypophysial hormones: stimulus-secretion coupling. In *Handbook of Physiology.* p 191-224. Section 7, Endocrinology, Volume IV. The Pituitary Gland and its Neuroendocrine Control Part I, eds RO Greep, EB Astwood, American Physiological Society, Washington, 1974.

Dousa TP. Interaction of lithium with vasopressin sensitive cyclic AMP system of human renal medulla. Endocrinology 95, 1359-1366, 1974.

Dousa T, Hechter O. The effect of Na Cl and Li Cl on vasopressin sensitive adenyl cyclases. Life Sci part I 9, 765-770, 1970.

Dreifuss JJ. A review on neurosecretory granules: their contents and mechanisms of release. Ann NY Acad Sci 248, 184-199, 1975.

Dreifuss JJ, Grau JD, Nordmann JJ. Calcium movements related to neurohypophysial hormone secretion. In *Calcium Transport in Contraction and Secretion.* pp 271-279, eds F Carafoli, F Clementi, W Drabikowski A Margreth, North-Holland Publishing Co, Amsterdam, 1975.

Dreifuss JJ, Kelly JS. The activity of identified supraoptic neurones and their responses to acetyl choline applied by iontophoresis. J Physiol Lond 220, 105-118, 1972.

Dreifuss JJ, Nordman JJ, Akert K, Sandri C, Moor H. Exo-endocytosis in the neurohypophysis as revealed by freeze-fracturing. In *Neurosecretion, The Final Neuroendocrine Pathway.* p 31-37, VI International Symposium, eds F Knowles, L Vollrath. Springer Verlag, New York, 1974.

Dudley HW. Some observations of the active principles of the pituitary gland. J Pharmacol 14, 295-312, 1919.

Dutton JW, Chin CJ, Hinchey EJ. The use of cholestyramine glucose solution to prevent vasopressin induced gastric erosions in pigs. J Surg Res 18, 501-504, 1975.

Du Vigneaud V. In *Les Prix Nobel en 1953* Stockholm, Kungl Bokt PA Norstedt and Soner, 1955.

Du Vigneaud V, Lawler HC, Popenoe EA. Enzymic cleavage of glycinamide from vasopressin and a proposed structure for this pressor antidiuretic of the posterior pituitary. J Am Chem Soc 75, 4480, 1953.

Dyball REJ, Henry JA. Relatively greater increase of oxytocin than vasopressin in the supra optic nucleus of rats after hypophysectomy. J Endocrinol 64, 125-131, 1975.

Dyckes DF, Nester JJ, Ferger MF, du Vigneaud V, Chan WY. (1-β-mercapto-β,β-diethylpropionic acid, 4-leucine) -8-lysine vasopressin and (1-β-mercapto-β,β-diethyl propionic acid, 4-leucine) oxytocin, compounds possessing antihormonal properties. J Med Chem 17, 969-972, 1974.

Earley LE, Martino JA, Friedler RM. Factors affecting sodium reabsorption by the proximal tubule as determined during blockade of distal sodium reabsorption. J Clin Invest 45, 1668-1684, 1966.

Edwards CRW, Chard T,Kitau MJ, Forsling ML, Landon J. The development of a radioimmunoassay for arginine vasopressin production of antisera and labelled hormone; separation techniques, specificity and sensitivity of the assay in aqueous solution. J Endocrinol 52, 279-288, 1972.

Eggena P, Christakis T, Deppisch L. Effect of hypotonicity on cyclic adenosine monophosphate formation and action in vasopressin target cells. Kidney Int 7, 161-169, 1975.

Eggena P, Schwartz IL, Walter R. Threshold and receptor reserve in the action of neurohypophysial peptides. A study of synergists and antagonists of the hydroosmotic response in toad urinary bladder. J Gen Physiol 56, 250-271, 1970.

Emilio MG, Menano HP. The excretion of hydrogen ion by the isolated amphibian skin: effects of amiloride and antidiuretic hormone. Biochim Biophys Acta 382, 344-352, 1975.

Epstein E, Pins DS, Miller M. Suppression of ADH during water immersion in normal man. J Appl Physiol 38, 1038-1044, 1975.

Errington ML, Rocha e Silva M. On the role of vasopressin and angiotensin in the development of irreversible haemorrhagic shock. J Physiol 242, 119-141, 1974.

Fabian MI. The metabolism of neurohypophysial hormones in mammals. Ph.D Thesis University of London, 1970.

Fabian MI, Forsling ML, Jones JJ, Pryor JS. The clearance and antidiuretic potency of neurohypophysial hormones in man and their plasma binding and stability. J Physiol 264, 653-668, 1969.

Farber MO, Bright TB, Strawbridge RA, Robertson GL, Manfredi F. Impaired water handling in chronic obstructive lung disease. J Lab Clin Med 85, 41-49, 1975.

Fehm HL, Voigt KH, Lang R. Characterisation of the CRF-like activity of vasopressin in vitro. Acta Endocrinol 78, Suppl 193, 129, 1975.

Ferguson DR, Twite BR. The effect of diuretics on Na^+, K^+-ATPase and cAMP levels in toad bladder epithelial cells. Naunyn Schmiedeberg's Arch Pharmacol 287, 111-116, 1975.

Fingeroth RT, Storer EH, Ramsby GR, Conn HO. Effect of intra-arterial infusion on hepatic artery flow. Surg Forum 24, 399-402, 1973.

Fisher CH, Sheff RN, Novak G, White RJ. The effect of superior mesenteric artery vasopressin infusions on cardiac output and coronary blood flow in dogs. Invest Radiol 9, 318, 1974.

Fitzsimons JT. Endocrine mechanisms in the control of water intake. In *Neural Integration of Physiological Mechanisms and Behaviour.* pp 226-247, eds GJ Mogenson, FR Calaresu, University of Toronto Press, Toronto and Buffalo, 1975.

Flament-Durand J, Dustin P. Action of colchicine on the neurosecretory paraventricular neurons in the rat. in *Neurosecretion, The Final Neuroendocrine Pathway.* p 304, VI International Symposium, eds F Knowles, L Vollrath, Springer Verlag, New York, 1974.

Flexner JB, Flexner LB, Hoffman PL, Walter R. Neurohypophyseal peptides and memory. Biophys J 15, 49a, 1975.

Flores J, Witkum P, Beckman B, Sharp WG. Reserve of vasopressin-sensitive adenylate cyclase in toad urinary bladder. Biochim Biophys Acta 362, 501-508, 1974.

Forn J. Lithium effects on the kidney. in *Lithium Research and Therapy.* pp 490-491, ed FN Johnson, Academic Press, New York, 1975.

Forrest JN, Cohen AD, Torretti J, Epstein FH. Lithium polyuria, an example of reversible nephrogenic diabetes insipidus. J Clin Invest 50, 32a, 1971.

Forsling ML - cited by AR Fuchs in *Endocrine Factors in Labour*, ed A Klopper, J Gardner, Cambridge University Press, 1973.

Forsling ML. Extraction of neurohypophysial hormones for bioassay. J Physiol Lond 241, 3-5P, 1974.

Forsling ML, Boyd NRH, Chard T. The dissociation of biological and immunological activity and biological activity of oxytocin: in vivo studies. In *Radioimmunoassay Methods*, eds KE Kirkham, WM Hunter, pp 549-555, Churchill Livingstone, Edinburgh and London, 1971.

Forsling ML, Ingram DM, Stanier MW. The effects of changes in hypothalamic temperature on ADH secretion in pigs. J Physiol Lond 247, 5-6P, 1975.

Forsling ML, Khokhar AM, Ramage CM, Slater JDH. Radioimmunoassay of arginine vasopressin in urine. J Physiol Lond 247, 5P, 1975.

Forsling ML, Martin MJ, Sturdy JC, Burton AM. Observations on the release and clearance of neurophysin and neurohypophysial hormones in the rat. J Endocrinol 57, 307-315, 1973.

Forsling ML, Rees M. Effects of hypoxia and hypercapnia on plasma vasopressin concentration. J Endocrinol 67, 62P-63P, 1975.

Forsling ML, Rheinhardt V, Himmler V. Neurohypophysial hormones and prolactin release. J Endocrinol 63, 579-580, 1974.

Forsling ML, Ullmann E. Release of vasopressin during hypoxia. J Physiol Lond 241, 35P-36P, 1974a.

Forsling ML, Ullmann E. Plasma vasopressin and renal concentrating ability in the anaesthetised dog. J Endocrinol 63, 41-42, 1974b.

Forsling ML, Ullmann E. Observations on oliguria in the anaesthetised dog. Kidney Int 8, 60, 1975a.

Forsling ML, Ullmann E. The effects of noradrenaline on the vasopressin concentration of plasma and on urine excretion in the dog. J Physiol Lond 247, 46P-47P, 1975b.

Frahm H, Smejkal E. Nachweir von ADH-Aktivitaten in Serum bei hypophysenperierten Patienten mit Polyurie und Kranken mit Diabetes Insipidus unter dem Einfluss eines antidiuretischen wirksamen psychotropen Antiepiliptikums (5 carbamyl-5H-dibenzo-carbam azepin = Tegretol). Verh Dtsch Gest Inn Med 75, 777-779, 1969.

Frazier LW. Inter-relationship of H^+ excretion and Na^+ reabsorption in toad urinary bladder. J Membr Biol 19, 267-276, 1974.

Fressinaud P, Carrol P, Menard J, Allegrini J. Radioimmunoassay of urinary antidiuretic hormone in man: stimulation suppression tests. Kidney Int 6, 184-190, 1974.

Fric I, Kodicek M, Flegel M, Zaoral M. Circular dichroic spectra of vasopressin analogues and their cyclic fragments. Eur J Biochem 56, 493-502, 1975.

Froger JL, Rofti J. Evolution du contenu en hormone antidiuretique de l'hypophyse chez le lapin nouveau-ne. CR Acad Sci (D), Paris 279, 1467-1470, 1974.

Furth AJ, Hope DB. Studies on the chemical modification of the tyrosine residue in bovine neurophysin II. Biochem J 116, 545-553, 1970.

Fukuchi S, Nakajima H, Takeuchi T, Nishizato K, Michimata Y. Measurement of plasma vasopressin by radioimmunoassay. Horuman To Rinsho 23, 85-90, 1975.

Fyhrquist F, Wallenius F. Improvement of antisera against polypeptide hormones. Nature 254, 82-83, 1975.

Fyro B, Sedvall G. Interaction of lithium with the elimination of electrolytes and fluid from the kidney. In *Lithium Research and Therapy*, pp 297-298, ed FN Johnson, Academic Press, New York, 1975.

Gagnon DJ, Cousineau D, Boucher PJ. Release of vasopressin by angiotensin II and prostaglandin E_2 from the rat neurohypophysis in vitro. Life Sci 12, 487-497, 1973.

Gagnon DJ, Sirois P, Park WK. Structural requirements for angiotensin analogues to accumulate cyclic AMP and release vasopressin from the incubated rat neurohypophysis. Clin Exp Pharmacol Physiol 2, 315-322, 1975.

Gagnon DJ, Sirois P, Boucher PJ. Stimulation by angiotensin II of the release of vasopressin from incubated rat neurohypophyses - possible involvement of cyclic AMP. Clin Exp Pharmacol Physiol 2, 305-313, 1975.

Garrud P. Effects of lysine-8-vasopressin on punishment-induced suppression of a lever-holding response. Prog in Brain Res 42, 173-186, 1975.

Geronilla DR, Sampliner JE, Lerner A. Gastrointestinal bleeding. Treatment with intra-arterial vasopressin. Am Surg 41, 321-326, 1975.

George CPL, Messerli FH, Genest J, Nowaczynski W, Boucher R, Kuchel O, Rojo-Ortega M. Diurnal variation of plasma vasopressin in man. J Clin Endocrinol Metab 41, 332-338, 1975.

Gilmore NJ, Vane JR. A sensitive and specific assay for vasopressin in circulating blood. Br J Pharmacol 38, 633-652, 1970.

Goetz KL, Bond GC, Bloxham DD. Atrial receptors and renal function. Physiol Rev 55, 157-205, 1975.

Goodman DBP, Bloom FE, Battenberg ER, Rasmussen H, Davis WL. Immunofluorescent localisation of cyclic AMP in toad urinary bladder: possible intercellular transfer. Science 188, 1023-1025, 1975.

Grainger F, Sloper JC. Overactivity of the hypothalamo-neurohypophysial neurosecretory system and the problem of the mechanisms of transporting neurosecretory material. in *Neurosecretion, The Final Neuroendocrine Pathway.* p 307, VI International Symposium, eds F Knowles, L Vollrath, Springer Verlag, New York, 1974.

Grantham JJ, Burg MB. Effect of vasopressin and cyclic AMP on permeability of isolated collecting tubules. Am J Physiol 211, 255-259, 1966.

Grantham JJ, Orloff J. Effect of prostaglandin E_1 on the permeability response of the isolated collecting tubule to vasopressin, adenosine 3', 5' monophosphate and theophylline. J Clin Invest 47, 1154-1161, 1968.

Gray LH, Conger AD, Ebert M, Hornsey S, Scott OCA. The concentration of oxygen dissolved in tissues at the time of irradiation as a factor in radiotherapy. Br J Radiol 26, 638-648, 1953.

Greenberg SR, Yudi M. Rapid reversal of inappropriate antidiuretic hormone secretion. Lancet i 547, 1971.

Grosso A, Spinelli F, De Sousa RC. The hydro-osmotic effect of vasopressin: a scanning electron microscope (SEM) study. Experientia 30, 679, 1974.

Guzek JW, Russell JT, Thorn NA. Inhibition by diphenylhydantoin of vasopressin from isolated rat neurohypophysis. Acta Pharmacol Toxicol Kbh 34, 1-4, 1974.

Hall D, Taylor A, Maffly R. Inhibition of vasopressin action by colchicine. Kidney Int 6, 49A, 1974.

Hall WJ, Martin JDG. Effect of calcium and vasopressin on the response of the frog skin to prostaglandin E_1. J Physiol Lond 240, 595-608, 1974.

Hamilton BP. Presence of neurophysin proteins in tumours associated with the syndrome of inappropriate ADH secretion. Ann NY Acad Sci 248, 153-156, 1975.

Hantman D, Rossier B, Zohlman R, Schrier R. Rapid correction of hyponatraemia in the syndrome of inappropriate secretion of antidiuretic hormone. Ann Intern Med 78, 870-875, 1973.

Hata N, Miura M. The inhibitory effect of the cerebellar fastigial stimulation on ADH secretion. J Physiol Lond 242, 793-803, 1974.

Hawker RW. Inactivation of antidiuretic hormone and oxytocin during pregnancy.

Quart J Exptl Physiol 41, 307-308, 1956.

Hayward JN. Neurohumoral regulation of neuroendocrine cells in the hypothalamus In *Recent Studies of Hypothalamic Function.* pp 166-179, Karger Basel, 1974.

Hayward JN. Effect of drugs of abuse on motivated behavior and magnocellular neuroendocrine cells. In *Narcotics and the Hypothalamus* pp 83-92, eds E Zimmerman and R George, Raven Press, New York, 1974.

Hayward JN, Barker MA. Diuretic and thermoregulatory response to preoptic cooling in the monkey. Am J Physiol 214, 843-850, 1968.

Hays RM, Levine SD. Vasopressin. Kidney Int 6, 307-322, 1974.

Heller H. The uteronic potency of vasopressin in the rat during the oestrus cycle and pregnancy. J Endocrinol 63, 42P, 1974.

Hems DA, Whitton PD. Stimulation by vasopressin of glycogen breakdown and gluconeogenesis in the perfused rat liver. Biochem J 136, 705-709, 1973.

Hems DA, Whitton PD, Gary MA. Metabolic actions of vasopressin, glycogon and adrenalin in the intact rat. Biochim Biophys Acta 411, 155-164, 1975.

Hewitt S, Debnam ES, Snart RS. Adrenal steroids and antidiuretic hormone action in toad bladder. J Endocrinol 65, 6P-7P, 1975.

Hiatt N, Miller A. Katayanagi T. Kaluresis and diuresis after administration of antidiuretic hormone to hyperkalemic dogs. Am J Physiol 228, 1108-1112, 1975.

Hillman SS. The effect of arginine vasopressin on water and sodium balance in the urodele amphibian *Aneides lugubris.* Gen Comp Endocrinol 24, 74-82, 1974.

Hochman S, Gutman Y.Lithium; ADH antagonism and ADH independent action in rats with diabetes insipidus. Eur J Pharmacol 28, 100-107, 1974.

Hoeg K, Andersen M. Lithiumfremkaldt diabetes insipidus pavirklig af anti-diuretisk hormon. Ugeskr laeger 137, 994-996,1975.

Hong JS, Poisner AM. Further studies on cold-induced release of vasopressin from isolated bovine neurosecretory granules. Neuroendocrinology 16, 165-177, 1974.

Hope DB. The neurophysin proteins: historical aspects. Ann NY Acad Sci 248, 6-14, 1975.

Hope DB, Pickup JC. Neurophysins. In *Handbook of Physiology*, pp 173-191, Section 7 Endocrinology, Vol 4. The Pituitary Gland and its Neuroendocrine Control, Part 1, eds RO Greep, EB Astwood, Amer Physiol Soc, Wash, 1974.

Hoppenstein JM, Miltenberger RW, Moran WH. The increase in blood levels of vasopressin in infants during birth and surgical procedures. Surg Gynecol Obstet 127, 966-974, 1968.

Hruby VJ, Spatola AF, Glasel JA, McKelvy JF. Equilibrium dialysis studies of hormone-neurophysin binding. Ann NY Acad Sci 248, 451-457, 1975.

Huang WC, Young TK. The absence of influence of oxytocin on the vasopressor action of arginine vasopressin in the rat. Clin J Physiol 21, 151-157, 1973.

Hui YSF, Barnes LD, Dousa TP. Effect of ethacrynic acid (EA) on enzymes related to cyclic AMP action in the renal medulla. Adv Cyclic Nucleotide Res 5, 818, 1975.

Huja BS, Szekerczes J, Hong SK. Effects of vasopressin on sodium transport across the toad skin. Kidney Int 6, 53A, 1974.

Hussain MK, Fernando N, Shapiro M, Kagan A, Glick SM. Radioimmunoassay of arginine vasopressin in human plasma. J Clin Endocrinol Metab 37, 616-625, 1973.

Imbert M, Chabardes D, Montegut M, Clique A, Morel F. Vasopressin dependent adenylate cyclase in single segments of rabbit kidney tubule. Pfluegers Arch 357, 173-186, 1975.

Imbert M, Chabardes D, Montegut M, Clique A, Morel F, Courrier MR. Presence d'une adenylate cyclase stimulee par la vasopressine dans la branche ascendante des anses des nephron du rein de lapin. C R Soc Biol Paris 280, 2129-2132, 1975.

Imbert M, Charbardes D, Morel F. Localisation et AVP target sites along the nephron: *Vth Int. Conf Nephrology*, C46, Florence, 1975.

Irmscher K, Sennejunker K, Wiegelman W, Solbach HG. Behandlung des Diabetes Insipidus mit 1, Desamino-8-D-arginin-vasopressin. Detche Med Wochenschr 99, 2431-2437, 1974.

Jacobson ED, Pawlick W, Mailman D, Burks T, Shepherd AP. Effects of vasoconstrictors on intestinal oxygen consumption. Gastroenterol 66, 715, 1974.

Jard S, Bockaert J. Stimulus-response coupling in neurohypophysial peptide target cells. Physiol Rev 55, 489-535, 1975.

Jard S, Roy C, Barth T, Rajerison R, Bockaert J. Antidiuretic hormone-sensitive kidney adenylate cyclase. Adv Cyclic Nucleotide Res 5, 31-52, 1975.

Jard S, Roy C, Rajerison R, Barth T, Bockaert J. Caracterisation du recepteur renal de l'hormone antidiuretique. J Urol Nephrol 80, 961-968, 1974.

Jenner FA, MacNeil S. Increased antidiuretic activity of rat urine following lithium activity. J Physiol Lond 245, 98P-99P, 1975.

Johnston CI, Hutchinson JS, Morris BJ, Dax EM. Release and clearance of neurophysins and posterior pituitary hormones. Ann NY Acad Sci 248, 272-279, 1975.

Jost K, Procazka Z, Cort JH, Barth T, Skopkova J, Prusik Z, Sorm F. Amino acids and peptides, CXXII. Synthesis and some biological activities of analogs of deaminovasopressin with the disulphide bridge altered to a tioether bridge. Collect Czech Chem Commun 39, 2835-2856, 1974.

Kappagoda CT, Linden RJ, Snow HM, Whitaker EM. Left atrial receptors and the antidiuretic hormone. J Physiol Lond 237, 663-683, 1974.

Katz B, Miledi R. A study of synaptic transmission in the absence of nerve impulses. J Physiol Lond 192, 407-426, 1967.

Kehne JH, Hughes FA, Gompertz ML. The use of surgical pituitrin in the control of oesophageal varix bleeding. Surgery 39, 917-925, 1956.

Keppens S, de Wulf H. Activation of liver glycogen phosphorylase by vasopressin. Arch Int Physiol Biochemie 82, 993-994, 1974.

Keppens S, de Wulf H. The action of liver glycogen phosphorylase by vasopressin. FEBS Letts 51, 29-32, 1975.

Keil LC, Summy-Long J, Severs WB. Release of vasopressin by angiotensin II. Endocrinology 96, 1063-1065, 1975.

Khokhar AM, Hough C, Slater JDH. Increased urine vasopressin concentration in essential hypertension. Clin Sci Mol Med 47, 9P, 1974.

Kilbinger H, Lohnes I, Muscholl E. Absence of muscarinic modulation of vasopressin release from the isolated rat neurohypophysis. Naunyn Schmiedebergs Arch Pharmacol 287, 391-398, 1975.

Kingsley DPE, Goldberg B, Abrahams C, Meyers A, Furman KI, Cohen I. Analgesic nephropathy. Brit Med J 4, 656, 1972.

Kirk CJ, Hems DA. Hepatic action of vasopressin; lack of a role for adenosine 3,5 cyclic monophosphate, FEBS Letts 47, 128-131, 1974.

Kirkham KE, Hunter WM - eds. *Radioimmunoassay Methods.* Churchill Livingstone, Edinburgh and London 1971 - Session III, Separation of bound from free labelled antigens, pp 243-342.

Kjessler B, Lundberg PO, Dysfunction of the neuroendocrine system in nine males with aspermia. Fertil Steril 25, 1007-1017, 1974.

Klassen NV, Purdie JW, Lynn KR, D'lorio M. Pulse radiolysis of oxytocin and lysine-vasopressin. Int J Radiat Biol 26, 127-132, 1974.

Knigge CM, Silverman AJ. Anatomy of the neuroendocrine hypothalamus. In *Handbook of Physiology*, pp 1-32, Section 7 Endocrinology, Vol 4. The Pituitary Gland and its neuroendocrine control Part I, eds RO Greep, EB Astwood. American Physiological Society, Wash, 1974.

Kozlowski S, Szczepanska-Sadowska E. Antagonistic effects of vasopressin and hypervolemia on osmotic reactivity of the thirst mechanism in dogs. Pfluegers Arch 353, 59-65, 1975.

Krisch B. Different populations of granules and their distribution in the hypothalamo-neurohypophysial tract of the rat under various experimental conditions. I Neurohypophysis, nucleus supraopticus and nucleus paraventricularis. Cell Tissue Res 151, 117-140, 1974.

Kuhn ER. Cholinergic and adrenergic release mechanism for vasopressin in the male rat: a study with injection of neurotransmitters and blocking agents into the third ventricle. Neuroendocrinology 16, 225-264, 1974.

Kurtzman NA, Boonjaren S. Physiology of antidiuretic hormone and the interrelationship between the hormone and the kidney. Nephron 167, 167-185, 1975.

Kurtzman NA, Rogers PW, Boonjaren S, Arruda JAL. Effect of infusion of pharmacologic amounts of vasopressin on renal electrolyte excretion. Am J Physiol 228, 890-894, 1975.

Kyncl J, Rudinger J. Excretion of antidiuretic activity in the urine of cats and rats after administration of the synthetic hormonogen N*α*glycl glycl glycl-(8-lysine)-vasopressin (triglycl vasopressin). J Endocrinol 48, 157, 1972.

Landolt AM. Treatment of acute post-operative inappropriate antidiuretic hormone secretion with diphenylhydantoin. Acta Endocrinol Kbh 76, 625-628, 1974.

Lauson HD. Metabolism of neurohypophysial hormones. In *Handbook of Physiology*, pp 287-396, Section 7 Endocrinology Vol 4. The Pituitary Gland and its Neuroendocrine Control Part 1, eds RO Greep, EB Astwood. American Physiological Society, Washington, 1974.

Laycock JF, Lee J, Lewis AF. The effect of chlorpromazine on water balance in pitressin-treated Brattleboro rats. Br J Pharmacol 52, 253-263, 1974.

Leaf A, Bartter FC, Santos RF, Wrong O. Evidence in man that urinary electrolyte loss induced by pitressin is a function of water retention. J Clin Invest 32, 868-878, 1953.

Lederis K. Neurosecretion and the functional structure of the neurohypophysis. In *Handbook of Physiology*, pp 81-102, Section 7 Endocrinology, Vol. IV, The Pituitary Gland and its Neuroendocrine Control, Part I, eds RO Greep, EB Astwood, American Physiological Society, Washington, 1974.

Lee J, DeWardener HE. Neurosecretion and sodium excretion. Kidney Int 6, 323-330, 1974.

Legros JJ. The radioimmunoassay of human neurophysins: contribution to the understanding of the pathophysiology of neurohypophysial function. Ann NY Acad Sci 248, 281-302, 1975.

Lindorf HH. Experimentelle Untersuchung der vascularen Wirkung von Adrenalin- und POR-8-Infiltration im Kieferbereich. Schweiz Monatsschr Zahnheilkd 85, 536-547, 1975.

Lishajko F, Andersson B. Recovery of ADH activity in the urine of goats under normal and stimulated conditions. Acta Physiol Scand 95, 102-109, 1975.

Little TM, Dowdle RH. Mycoplasma pneumonia with inappropriate secretion of antidiuretic hormone. Br Med J 1, 517, 1975.

Livett BG. Immunochemical studies on the storage and oxonal transport of neurophysins in the hypothalamo-neurohypophysial system. Ann NY Acad Sci 248, 112-132, 1975.

MacFarlane DE, Mills DCB. The effects of ATP on platelets: evidence against the central role of released ADP in primary aggregation. Blood 46, 309-320, 1975.

McKelvy JF. Phosphorylation of neurosecretory granules by cAMP-stimulated protein kinase and its implication for the transport and release of neurophysin proteins. Ann NY Acad Sci 248, 80-91, 1975.

McNeill JR, Stark RD, Greenway CV. Intestinal vasoconstriction after haemorrhage: roles of vasopressin and angiotensin. Am J Physiol 219, 1342-1347, 1970.

McNeill JR. Intestinal vasoconstriction following diuretic-induced volume depletion: role of angiotensin and vasopressin. Can J Physiol Pharmacol 52, 829-839, 1974.

MacNeil S, Jenner FA. Lithium and polyuria. in *Lithium Research and Therapy*, pp 473-484, ed FN Johnson, Academic Press, NY, 1975.

Magnus R, Schafer EA. The action of pituitary extracts upon the kidney. J Physiol Lond 27, ix-x, 1901.

Mandel LJ. Actions of external hypertonic urea, ADH and theophylline on transcellular and extracellular solute permeabilities in frog skin. J Gen Physiol 65, 599-616, 1975.

Manning M, Balaspiri L, Judd J, Acosta M, Sawyer WH. Probing the molecular basis of antidiuretic specificity and duration of action with synthetic peptides. FEBS Lett 44, 229-232, 1974.

Mannucci PM. Enhancement of plasminogen activator by vasopressin and adrenaline - a role of cyclic AMP. Thromb Res 4, 539-549, 1974.

Mannucci PM, Pareti FI, Barbi GL. Effect of cyclic AMP and related drugs on plasminogen activator. In *Synthetic and Thrombolytic Agents: Chemical, Biochemical, Pharmacological and Clinical Aspects, pp* 402-409, Proc 1st Int Symp, Paris, eds KN Von Kaulla, JF Davidson, CC Thomas, Springfield, Ill, 1975.

Mannucci PM, Pareti O, Barbi GL. Effect of cyclic AMP and related drugs on plasminogen activator. Abstract from First Symposium on Synthetic Fibrinolytic Agents, Paris, 1972.

Markoff N, Hobl E, Horder MH, Flury A, Ratti R. Erste Erfahrungen mit der intra arteriellen not fallmassigen octapressin - Therapie der massive oberen Magen-Darm-Blutung. Z. Gastroenterol 11, 307-312, 1973.

Marks BH, Sakai KK, George JM, Koestner A. A new technique for studying neuroendocrine systems. In *Narcotics and the Hypothalamus*, pp 95-108, eds E Zimmerman and R George, Raven Press, NY, 1974.

Martinez-Maldonado M, Stavroulaki-Tsapara A, Tsaparas N, Suki WN, Eknoyan G. Renal effects of lithium administration in rats: Alterations in water and electrolyte metabolism and the response to vasopressin and cyclic-adenosine monophosphate during prolonged administration. J Lab Clin Med 86,445-461, 1975.

Masur SK, Holtzman E, Walter R. Hormone-stimulated exocytosis in the toad urinary bladder. Some possible implications for turnover of surface membranes. J Cell Biol 52, 211-219, 1972.

Meinders AE, Cejka V, Robertson GL. The antidiuretic action of carbamazapine in man. Clin Sci Mol Med 47, 289-299, 1974.

Meienhofer J, Trzeciak A, Dousa T, Hechter O, Havran RJ, Schwartz IL, Walter R. Solid phase synthesis and some pharmacological properties of 8-arginine vasopressin and 8-arginine vasopressinoic acid. In *Peptides*, pp 157-159, North Holland Publishing, 1969.

Merrifield RB. The synthesis of a tetrapeptide. Am J Chem Soc 85, 2149-2154, 1963.

Meyer-Grass M, Pliska V. Properties of neurophysin from neurosecretory granules ("native" neurophysin?). Experientia 30, 689, 1974.

Miller AM, Moses M. Radioimmunoassay of urinary antidiuretic hormone with application to study of the Brattleboro rat. Endocrinology 88, 1397-1396, 1971.

Miller AM, Moses M. Urinary antidiuretic hormone in polyuric disorders and inappropriate ADH syndrome. Ann Intern Med 77, 715-721, 1972.

Miller AM, Moses M. Radioimmunoassay of urinary antidiuretic hormone in man: Response to water load and dehydration in normal subjects. J Clin Endocrinol Metab 34, 537-545, 1972.

Millette B, Huet PM, Lavoie P, Viallet A. Portal and systemic effects of selective infusion of vasopressin into the superior mesenteric artery in cirrhotic patients. Gastroenterology 69, 6-12, 1975.

Milton AS, Paterson A. Microinjection study of the role of adrenergic transmission in the control of secretion of antidiuretic hormone. Br J Pharmacol 43, 444P-445P, 1971.

Minchin MCW, Nordmann JJ. The release of ^{3}H gamma-aminobutyric acid and neurophysin from the isolated rat posterior pituitary. Brain Res 90, 75-84, 1975.

Mirsky IA. Relative effects of insulin oxytocin and vasopressin on free fatty acid concentration of the plasma of non-diabetic and diabetic dogs. Endocrinology 73, 613-618, 1963.

Mitrovic M, Ristic B. Our experience in local vasoconstrictor POR-8 in surgical oto-rhino-laryngology. Srpski Arhiv Za Tselokupno Lekarstvo 102, 591-598, 1974.

Mohring J, Mohring B, Schomig A, Schomig-Breckner H, Haack D. Acute effects of vasopressin on potassium and water balance in rats with diabetes insipidus. Am J Physiol 227, 921-926, 1974.

Molnarova B, Sova O. The influence of pH in the medium on the degradation of neural hormones by pregnancy serum. Physiol Bohemoslov 24, (3), 199-208, 1975.

Mor J, Ben-Galim E, Abrahamov A. Inappropriate antidiuretic hormone production in an infant with severe pneumonia. Am J Dis Child 129, 133-135, 1975.

Moran WH, Miltenberger FW, Shuayb WA, Zimmerman B. The relationship of antidiuretic hormone to surgical stress. Surgery 56, 99-108, 1964.

Morgan ML, Akatsuka N, Wilson MF, Moran WH, Sizemore A. Renal blood flow and intrarenal flow distribution with steady state plasma vasopressin levels. Fed Proc 34, 364, 1975.

Morton JJ, Padfield PL, Forsling ML. A radioimmunoassay for plasma arginine-vasopressin in man and dog: application to physiological and pathological states. J Endocrinol 65, 411-424, 1975.

Morton JJ, Waite MA. The possible relationship between the affinity of arginine vasopressin antibodies and the degree of polyuria and polydipsia in actively immunized rabbits. J Endocrinol 54, 523-524, 1972.

Moses M, Miller AM. Osmotic influences on the release of vasopressin. In *Handbook of Physiology*, pp 225-242, Section 7 Endocrinology, Vol 4. The Pituitary Gland and its Neuroendocrine Control Part I, eds RO Greep, EB Astwood. Amer. Physiological Society, Washington 1974.

Moses M, Miller AM. Drug-induced dilutional hyponatremia. New Engl J Med 291, 1234-1239, 1974.

Moses M, van Gemert M, Miller AM. Evidence that glyburide-induced diuresis is not mediated by inhibition of ADH. Horm Res 5, 359-366, 1974.

Moss RL, Dyball REJ, Cross BA. Responses of antidromically identified supraoptic and paraventricular units to acetylcholine, noradrenaline and glutamate applied iontophoretically. Brain Res 35, 573-575, 1971.

Muller JR, Thorn NA, Torp-Pedersen C. Effects of calcium and sodium on vasopressin release in vitro induced by a prolonged potassium stimulation.Acta Endocrinol Kbh 79, 51-59, 1975.

Munoz O, Valencia R, Lopez E, Junco E. Secrecion desordenada de hormona Antidiuretica en infecciones del sistema nervosa central. Bol Med Hosp Infant Mex 32, 13-24, 1975.

Musky IA. Effects of oxytocin, vasopressin and related peptides on plasma FFA of non-diabetic and diabetic dogs. Am J Physiol 204, 842-846, 1963.

Myers JB. Inappropriate ADH secretion in chest disease. Br Med J 3, 785-787, 1974.

Naftalin L. Hormonal control of water and electrolytes. Otolaryngol Clin NA 8, 293-301, 1975.

Nagasubramanian S. The effect of vasopressin on the facility of aqueous humour outflow in the rabbit. Ophthalmic Res 6 301-307, 1974.

Nakano J. Cardiovascular effect of oxytocin in rodents and a marsupial. Proc Soc Exp Biol Med 115, 707-709, 1964.

Nardacci NJ, Mukhopadhyay S, Campbell BJ. Partial purification and characterisation of the antidiuretic hormone-inactivating enzyme from renal plasma membranes. Biochim Biophys Acta 377, 146-157, 1975.

Nemethova V, Lichardus B. Clinical experience with DDAVP (1-deamino-8-D-arginine vasopressin) in the treatment of diabetes insipidus in children. Endokrinologie 63, 137-141, 1974.

Nestor JJ, Ferger MF. (4-phenyl alanine) oxytocin as an inhibitor of the antidiuretic effect of 8 arginine vasopressin. J Med Chem 18, 1022-1024, 1975.

Nordmann JJ. Hormone release in relation to inactivation of Ca-entry in the rat neurohypophysis. J Physiol Lond 249, 38-39P, 1975.

Nordmann JJ. Hormone release and Ca uptake in the rat neurohypophysis. In *Calcium Transport in Contraction and Secretion.* pp 281-286, eds F Carafoli, F Clementi, W Drabikowski, North Holland Publishing Co, 1975.

Nordmann JJ, Currell GA. The mechanism of calcium ionophore induced secretion from the rat neurohypophysis. Nature 253, 646-647, 1975.

Norstrom A. The heterogeneity of the neurohypophysial pool of neurophysin. In *Neurosecretion, the Final Neuroendocrine Pathway.* VI International Symposium, eds F Knowles, L Vollrath, Springer Verlag, NY, 1974.

Norstrom A. Axonal transport and turnover of neurohypophyseal hormones in the rat. Ann NY Acad Sci 248, 46-62, 1975.

Norstrom A, Sjostrand J. Axonal transport of proteins in the hypothalamo-neurohypophysial system of the rat. J Neurochem 18, 29-39, 1971.

Novich RK. Drug-induced dilutional hyponatraemia. N Engl J Med 292, 716-717, 1975.

Nusbaum M, Baum S, Sakiyalak P, Blakemore C. Pharmacologic control of portal hypertension. Surgery 62, 299-310, 1967.

Nusbaum M, Conn HO. Arterial vasopressin infusions: science or sceance? Gastroenterology 69, 263-267, 1975.

O'Connor WJ. *Renal Function.* Edward Arnold, London (pp 58-59), 1962.

Ohno T, Goodman DPB, Rasmussen H, Omura S. A new type of sodium transport inhibitor on the toad bladder. J Membr Biol 18, 295-304, 1974.

Olivecrona H. Paraventricular nucleus and pituitary gland. Acta Physiol Scan 40, Suppl 136, 1-178, 1957.

Oliver G, Schafer EA. On the physiological action of extracts of the pituitary body and certain other glandular organs. J Physiol Lond 18, 277-279, 1895.

Olsson K, Kolmodin R. Inhibition of antidiuretic hormone secretion by intracarotid infusions of slightly hypertonic non-electrolyte solutions. Acta Endocrinol 76, 53-58, 1974.

Orloff J, Handler JS, Stoff JS. Permissive effect of aldosterone on the action of vasopressin. Alferd Benzon Symp 5, 205-213, 1973.

Oyama SN, Kagan A, Glick SM. Radioimmunoassay of vasopressin: application to unextracted human urine. J Clin Endocrinol 33, 739-744, 1971.

Park YS, Hong SK. Solomon S. Interaction of amphotericin B and vasopressin in toad urinary bladder and rat nephron. Fed Proc 34, 270, 1975.

Parkin JM. DDAVP in diabetes insipidus. Arch Dis Chid 50, 84, 1975.

Pearson DB, Goodman R, Sachs H. Stimulated vasopressin synthesis by a foetal hypothalamic factor. Science 187, 1081-1082, 1975.

Pearson D, Shainberg A, Osinchak J, Sachs H. The hypothalamo-neurohypophysial complex in organ culture: Morphologic and biochemical characteristics. Endocrinology 96, 982-993, 1975.

Peck JW, Blass EM. Localisation of thirst and antidiuretic osmoreceptors by intracranial injections in rats. Am J Physiol 228, 1501-1509, 1975.

Peptide Hormone Group. Shanghai Institute of Biochemistry. An improved solid-phase method for peptide synthesis - the synthesis of oxytocin and vasopressin. Scientica Sinica 18, 233-241, 1975.

Perks AM, Vizsolyi E. Studies of neurohypophysial peptides during foetal life. In *Neurosecretion, The Final Common Pathway.* p 317, VIth International Symposium London, eds F Knowles, L Vollrath, Springer Verlag, NY, 1974.

Perris AD, Hunt NH. Stimulation of mitosis in rat bone marrow cells by antidiuretic hormone after haemorrhage. J Endocrinol 65, 5-6P, 1975.

Petrucelli RJ, Eggena P. Effect of vasopressin on urea and thiourea transport across the toad bladder. C236, Proc Vth Int. Conf Nephrology, Florence, 1975.

Philbin DM, Baratz RA, Patterson RW. The effect of carbon dioxide on plasma antidiuretic hormone levels during intermittent positive pressure breathing. Anaesthesiology 33, 345-349, 1970.

Pietras RJ, Seeler BJ, Szego CM. Influence of antidiuretic hormone on release of lysosomal hydrolase at mucosal surface of epithelial cells from urinary bladder. Nature 257, 493-495, 1975.

Pickering BT, Jones CW. Isolation of labelled neurohypophysial hormones from rat neural lobes after the intra cisternal injection of (3H) tyrosine. J Endocrinol 46, VI, 1970.

Pickering BT, Jones CW, Burford GD. Biochemical aspects of the hypothalamo-neurohypophysial neurone. In *Neurosecretion, The Final Neuroendocrine Pathway*, pp 72-85, VI International Symposium, eds F Knowles, L Vollrath, Springer Verlag, NY, 1974.

Pickering BT, Jones CW, Burford GD, McPherson M, Swann RW, Heap PR, Morris JF. The role of neurophysin proteins: suggesting from the study of their transport and turnover. Ann NY Acad Sci 248, 15-35, 1975.

Pliska V. Heterogeneous binding sites in neurophysin-like macromolecules; some theoretical and computational considerations. Ann NY Acad Sci 248, 480-493, 1975.

Pliska V, Meyer-Grass M. Some properties of neurophysin isolated from bovine neurosecretory granules. Ann NY Acad Sci 248, 235-245, 1975.

Pliska V, Meyer-Grass M, Sunde D. Binding protein from neurosecretory granules with high affinity for vasopressin ("native" neurophysin?). In *Neurosecretion, The Final Neuroendocrine Pathway*, p 319, VI International Symposium, eds F. Knowles, L Vollrath, Springer Verlag, NY, 1974.

Poisner AM, Hong JS. Storage and release of vasopressin from neurosecretory granules and the neurohypophysis. In *Advances in Cytopharmacology,* pp 303-310, eds B Ceccarelli, F Clementi, J Meldolesi, Raven Press, NY, 1974.

Porter JC, Ben-Jonathan N, Oliver C, Eskay RL. Secretion of releasing hormones from CSF to hypophysial portal blood. In *Brain-Endocrine Interaction II.* pp 295-305, The Ventricular System, 2nd Int Symp, Shizoka, Karger, Basel, 1975.

Rado JP. Evidence for permanent enhancement of residual ADH induced by antidiuretic agents (chlorpropamide, carbamazepine, clofibrate) in patients with pituitary diabetes insipidus. Endokrinologie 64, 217-222, 1975.

Rado JP, Borbely L, Szende L, Tako J. Decreased antidiuretic response to lysine-vasopressin after acute administration of gibenclamide in healthy subjects. Acta Diabetol Lat 11, 18-25, 1974.

Radomski JL, Fuyat HN, Nelson AA, Smith PA. The toxic effects, excretion and distribution of lithium chloride. J Pharmacol Exp Ther 100, 421-444, 1950.

Raij K, Harkonen M, Mulder J, Aldercreutz H. Effect of the carboxyl-terminal tripeptide of vasopressin on plasma free fatty acids and cyclic adenosine monophosphate in man. Scand J Lab Clin Invest 35, 253-257, 1975.

Raij K, Perheentupa J, Harkonen M. Urinary cyclic adenosine monophosphate excretion in diabetes insipidus of childhood. Scand J Lab Clin Invest 34, 177-184, 1974.

Rappleye AT, Johnson GH, Olsen JD, Lagasse LD. The radioprotective effects of vasopressin on the gastro-intestinal tract of mice. Radiology 117, 199-203, 1975.

Raskind MA, Orenstein H, Christopher TG. Acute psychosis, increased water ingestion and inappropriate antidiuretic hormone secretion. Am J Psychiatry 132, 907-910, 1975.

Rasmussen H, Schwartz IL, Young R, Marc-Aurele JM. Structural requirements for the action of neurohypophysial hormones upon the isolated amphibian urinary membrane. J Gen Physiol 46, 1171-1189, 1963.

Ratnikov VI. Changes produced by analgesics in the sensitivity of the kidneys to antidiuretic hormone. Biull Eksp Biol Med 79, 63-65, 1975.

Rayson B, Morgan T. Interrelationship between antidiuretic hormone, adenyl cyclase, cyclic AMP and water permeability. In *Proc Vth Int. Conf Nephrology,*

C191, Florence, 1975.

Reed PW, Lardy HA. A23187: a divalent cation ionophore. J Biol Chem 247, 6970-6977, 1972.

Reed S, Beck N. Effect of potassium (K) depletion (↓) on vasopressin (VP) dependent cyclic AMP (cAMP) system in rat renal medulla (RRM). Adv Cyclic Nucleotide Res 5, 817, 1975.

Rees LH, Ratcliffe JG. Ectopic hormone production by non-endocrine tumours. Clin Endocrinol Oxf 3, 263-299, 1974.

Reinharz A, Vallotton MB. Presence of peptidase in bovine pineal gland. Experientia 30, 691, 1974.

Rich DH, Gesseellchen PD, Tong A, Cheung A, Buckner CK. Alkylating derivatives of amino acids and peptides: Synthesis of **N**-maleoylamino acids, (1-[**N**-maleoylglycyl) cysteinyl] oxytocin and (1-[**N**-maleoyl-11-aminoundecanoyl] cysteinyl) oxytocin. Effects on vasopressin-stimulated water loss from isolated toad bladder. J Med Chem 18, 1004-1010, 1975.

Rigter H, Riezen H van, Wied D de. Effects of ACTH and vasopressin analogues on CO_2-induced retrograde amnesia in rats. Physiol Behav 13, 381-388, 1974.

Rist E. Treatment of haemoptysis by intravenous injection of pituitrin. Bull Mem Hosp, Paris 1, 776, 1913. Cited by Geronilla, Sampliner, Lerner, 1975.

Ritter RJ, Tucker RE, Schelling GT, Mitchell GE. Renal response to vasopressin infusion in vitamin A-deficient and normal ewes. J Anim Sci 40, 103-107, 1975.

Roache MR. A biophysical look at the relation of structure and function in the umbilicus. In *Foetal and Neonatal Physiology.* pp 141-163, Proc of the Sir Joseph Barcroft Centenary Symposium. Cambridge Univ. Press, London, 1973.

Robertson GL. Vasopressin in osmotic regulation in man. Ann Rev Med 25, 345-322, 1974.

Robertson GL, Bhoopalam N, Zelkowitz LJ. Vincristine neurotoxicity and abnormal secretion of antidiuretic hormone. Arch Intern Med 132, 717-720, 1973.

Robertson GL, Klein LA, Roth J, Gorden P. Immunoassay of plasma vasopressin in man. Proc Nat Acad Sci USA 66, 1298-1305, 1970.

Robertson GL, Mahr EA, Athar S, Sinha T. Development and clinical application of a new method for the radioimmunoassay of arginine vasopressin in human plasma. J Clin Invest 52, 2340-2352, 1973.

Robinson AG. Radioimmunoassay of neurophysin proteins: utilisation of specific neurophysin assays to demonstate independent secretion of different neurophysins in vivo. Ann NY Acad Sci 248, 246-254, 1975.

Robinson AG, Zimmerman EA. Cerebrospinal fluid and ependymal neurophysin. J Clin Invest 52, 1260-1267, 1973.

Rocha AS, Kokko JP. Permeability of medullary nephron segments to urea and water: effect of vasopressin. Kidney Int 6, 379-387, 1974.

Rocha e Silva M, Rosenberg M. The release of vasopressin in response to haemorrhage and its role in the mechanism of blood pressure regulation. J Physiol Lond 202, 535-557, 1969.

Rosenbloom AA, Fisher DA. Radioimmunoassayable AVT and AVP in adult mammalian brain tissue: comparison of normal and Brattleboro rats. Neuroendocrinology 17, 354-361, 1975.

Roy C. Characterisation of the renal antidiuretic hormone receptor: relations of hormone binding to adenylate cyclase activation. In *INSERM Colloquium*, p 190, Physiologie du Nephron, Mecanismes et Regulation, 1974.

Roy C, Barth T, Jard S. Vasopressin-sensitive kidney adenylate cyclase. Structural requirements for attachment to the receptor and enzyme activation studies with vasopressin analogues. J Biol Chem 250, 3149-3156, 1975.

Roy J, Havran RT, Schwartz IL, Walter R. Oxytocin analogs with substitutions in positions 3 and 4. Synthesis and some pharmacological properties. Int J Peptide Protein Res 7, 171-178, 1975.

Roy C, Rajerison J, Bockaert J, Jard S. Solubilisation of the renal antidiuretic hormone receptor. Adv Cyclic Nucleotide Res 5, 811, 1975.

Rubin MS. Chemical modification of vasopressin induced transport across toad bladder. Fed Proc 34, 327, 1975.

Ruch W. Estimation of antidiuretic hormone in the urine of healthy subjects and patients with inappropriate secretion of vasopressin (Schwartz, Bartter syndrome) Acta Endocrinol Kbh 54, 113-121, 1967.

Ruoff HJ, Gosbee JL, Lederis K. Substances affecting the release of neurohypophysial hormones. In *Recent Studies of Hypothalamic Function.* pp 67-79, Int Symp Calgary, Karger, Basel, 1974.

Russell JT, Hansen EL, Thorn NA. Calcium and stimulus-secretion coupling in the neurohypophysis, III. Ca^{2+} ionophore (A23187)-induced release of vasopressin from isolated rat neurohypophyses. Acta Endocrinol Kbh. 77, 443-450, 1974.

Russell JT, Thorn NA. Calcium and stimulus-secretion coupling in the neurohypophysis. In *Neurosecretion, The Final Neuroendocrine Pathway,* p 321, VI International Symposium, eds F. Knowles, L Vollrath, Springer Verlag, New York, 1974.

Russell JT, Thorn NA. Adenosine triphosphate dependent calcium uptake by subcellular fractions from bovine neurohypophyses. Acta Physiol Scand 93, 364-377, 1975.

Russell JT, Warberg J, Thorn NA. Calcium and stimulus-secretion coupling in the neurohypophysis. IV. Effect of N-ethylmaleimide on $^{45}Ca^{2+}$ transport and vasopressin release by isolated rat neurohypophyses. Acta Endocrinol Kbh 77, 691-698, 1974.

Rutsky EA. Inappropriate secretion of antidiuretic hormone. South Med J 68,

59-64, 1975.

Sadowski J, Kurkus J, Chwalbinska-Moneta J. Plasma hormone and renal function changes in unrestrained dogs exposed to cold. Am J Physiol 228, 376-381, 1975.

Saffran M, Pearlmutter AF, Rapino E. Upton GV. Pressinoic acid: a peptide with potent corticotrophin-releasing activity. Biochem Biophys Res Commun 48, 748-751, 1972.

Sakai KK, Marks BH, George JM, Koestner A. The isolated organ-cultured supra-optic nucleus as a neuropharmacological test system. J Pharmacol Exp Ther 190, 482-491, 1974.

Sawyer WH. The mammalian antidiuretic response. In *Handbook of Physiology.* pp 443-468, Section 7 Endocrinology, Vol 4. The Pituitary Gland and its Neuro-endocrine Control Part I, eds RO Greep, EB Astwood, American Physiological Society, Washington, 1974.

Sawyer CH, Gernandt BE. Effects of intracarotid and intraventricular injections of hypertonic solutions on electrical activity of the rabbit brain. Am J Physiol 185, 209-216, 1956.

Scharrer E. Neurosecretion in the vertebrates; a survey. Publ Statz zool Napoli 24, Suppl Convegno sulla Neurosecrezione, pp 18-20, 1954.

Scheiner E. The relationship of antidiuretic hormone to the control of volume and tonicity in the human. Adv Clin Chem 17, 1-52, 1975.

Schmid FG, Abboud FM, Wendling MG, Ramberg ES, Mark AL, Heistad RD, Eckstein JW. Regional vascular effects of vasopressin: plasma levels and circulatory responses. Am J Physiol 227, 998-1004, 1974.

Schneck SA, von Kaulla KN. Fibrinolysis and the nervous system. Neurology 11, 959-969, 1961.

Schorn D. Inappropriate antidiuretic hormone secretion: two cases presenting with pulmonary tuberculosis. S Afr Med J 48, 1161-1162, 1974.

Schrier RW. Effects of adrenergic nervous system and catecholamines on renal hemodynamic, sodium and water excretion and renin secretion. Kidney Int 6, 291-306, 1974.

Schrier RW, Berl T. Mechanism of effect of β-adrenergic stimulation with norepinephrine on renal water excretion. J Clin Invest 52, 97-111, 1973.

Schrier RW, Berl T. Nonosmolar factors affecting renal water excretion. N Engl J Med 292, 81-88, 1975.

Schrier RW, Berl T. Harbottle JA, McDonald KM. Catecholamines and renal water excretion. Nephron 15, 186-196, 1975.

Schrier RW, Reid IA, Berl T, Earley LE. Parasympathetic pathways, renin secretion and vasopressin release. Clin Sci Mol Med 48, 83-89, 1975.

Schwartz WB, Bennet W, Curelop G, Bartter FC. The syndrome of renal sodium loss and hyponatraemia probably resulting from inappropriate secretion of antidiuretic hormone. Am J Med 23, 529-542, 1957.

Schwartz IL, Walter R. Neurohypophyseal hormone-calcium inter-relationships in the toad bladder. In *Protein and Polypeptide Hormones*, pp 264-269, ed M Margoulies, Amsterdam, Excerpta Medical Foundation, 1968.

Scott WN, Saperstein VS, Yoder MJ. Partition of tissue functions in epithelia: localisation of enzymes in mitochondria-rich cells of toad urinary bladder. Science 184, 797-799, 1974.

Sedlakova E, Kluh I, Barth T, Jost K. Neurophysin binding of some analogs of neurohypophysial hormones. Collect Czechoslav Chem Comm 39, 2988-3002, 1974.

Segar WE, Moore WW. The regulation of antidiuretic hormone release in man. Effects of changes in posture and ambient temperature on blood ADH levels. J Clin Invest 47, 2143-2151, 1968.

Shade RE, Share L. Vasopressin release during nonhypotensive hemorrhage and angiotensin II infusion. Am J Physiol 228, 149-154, 1975.

Share L. Acute reduction in extracellular fluid volume and the concentration of antidiuretic hormone in blood. Endocrinology 69, 925-933, 1961.

Share L. Blood pressure, blood volume and the release of vasopressin. In *Handbook of Physiology*, pp 243-256, Section 7 Endocrinology, Vol 4, eds RO Greep, EB Astwood. American Physiological Society, Washington, 1974.

Sharp WG, Leaf A. Mechanisms of action of aldosterone. Physiol Rev 46, 593-633, 1966.

Shute CCD, Lewis PR. Cholinergic and monoaminergic pathways in the hypothalamus. Br Med Bull 22, 221-226, 1966.

Silverman AJ, Knigge KM, Zimmerman EA. Ultrastructural immunocytochemical localisation of neurophysin in freeze-substituted neurohypophysis. Am J Anat 142, 265-271, 1975.

Silverman AJ, Kozlowski GP, Zimmerman EA. Ultrastructural immunocytochemical localisation of neurophysin (NP) and vasopressin (VP) in the neural lobe and median eminence of guinea pig. Anat Rec 181, 479-480, 1975.

Silverman AJ, Zimmerman EA. Ultrastructural immunocytochemical localisation of neurophysin and vasopressin in the median eminence and posterior pituitary of the guinea pig. Cell Tissue Res 159, 291-301, 1975.

Singer I, Franko EA. Lithium induced ADH resistance in toad urinary bladders. Kidney Int 3, 151-159, 1973.

Singh I, Malhotra MS, Khanna PK, Nanda RB, Purshottam T, Upadhyay TN, Radhakrishnan O, Brahmachari HD. Changes in plasma cortisol, blood antidiuretic hormone and urinary catecholamines in high altitude pulmonary oedema. Int J Biometeorol 18, 211-221, 1974.

Sirinek KR, Thomford NR. Pharmacological control of post-hepatectomy portal hypotension. Surg Forum 24, 391-393, 1973.

Sirinek KR, Thomford NR. The hemodynamic response of cirrhotic patients to the combined administration of vasopressin and isoproterenol. Rev Surg 32, 217-220, 1975a.

Sirinek KR, Thomford NR. Isoproterenol in offsetting adverse effects of vasopressin in cirrhotic patients. Am J Surg 129, 130-136, 1975b.

Sjostrand T. The regulation of the blood distribution in man. Acta Physiol Scand 26, 312-327, 1952.

Skowsky WR, Bashore RA, Smith FG, Fisher DA. In *Foetal and Neonatal Physiology*, pp 439-447, Proc. of the Sir Joseph Barcroft Centenary Symposium. Cambridge Univ. Press, London, 1973.

Skowsky WR, Rosenbloom AA, Fisher DA. Radioimmunoassay measurement of arginine vasopressin in serum: development and application. J Clin Endocrinol Metab 37, 278-287, 1974.

Slepushkin VD. The effect of vasopressin on excretion of magnesium and other electrolytes. Fiziol Zh SSSR 61, 279-283, 1975.

Small CW, Watkins WB. Glutathione-oxytocin transhydrogenase of human placental origin with specificity towards neurohypophysial hormones. Nature 251, 237-239, 1974.

Smith CW, Clark W, Ferger MF, Chan WY. Synthesis and some pharmacological properties of [3-2-thienyl)-L-alanine]-8-lysine-vasopressin. J Med Chem 18, 822-825, 1975.

Smith HW. Renal excretion of sodium and water. Fed Proc 11, 701-705, 1952.

Somlyo AP, Somlyo AV. Vascular smooth muscle II. Pharmacology of normal and hypertensive vessels. Pharmacol Rev 22, 249-253, 1970.

Solovera LP. Methods of determination of antidiuretic hormone in blood. Kardiologia 15, 147-148, 1975.

Spanos A, Spry J. Inappropriate secretion of antidiuretic hormone with chronic chest infection. Br Med J 3, 785-786, 1974.

Spinelli F, Grosso A, De Sousa RC. Effects of vasopressin and cytochalasin B on apical membranes of toad bladder and collecting duct in the mammalian kidney. In *INSERM Colloquium,* Physiologie du Nephron, p195, Mecanismes et Regulation, 1974.

Stuart MJ, Cuaso C, Miller M, Oski FA. Syndrome of recurrent increased secretion of antidiuretic hormone following multiple doses of vincristine. Blood 45, 315-370, 1975.

Stutinsky F. Morphological and physiological reactions of the supraoptic and paraventricular nuclei. In *Neurosecretion, the Final Neuroendocrine Pathway.* pp 15-23, eds F Knowles and L Vollrath, Springer-Verlag, NY, 1974.

Svenningsen MW, Aronson AS. Post natal development of renal concentrating capacity as estimated by DDAVP-test in normal and asphyxiated neonates. Biol Neonate 25, 230-241, 1974.

Szczepanska-Sadowska E. Plasma ADH increase and thirst suppression elicited by pre-optic heating in the dog. Am J Physiol 226, 155-161, 1974.

Szczepanska-Sadowska E, Kozlowski S, Sobocinska J. Blood antidiuretic hormone level and osmotic reactivity of thirst mechanism in dogs. Am J Physiol 227, 766-770, 1974.

Taylor A, Maffly R, Wilson L, Reaven E. Evidence for involvement of microtubules in the action of vasopressin. Ann NY Acad Sci 253, 723-737, 1975.

Taylor A, Reaven E. Microtubule content of toad bladder epithelial cells: effect of colchicine and vasopressin. *Proc Vth Int Conf Nephrology,* C143, Florence, 1975.

Thomford NR, Sirinek KR. Intravenous vasopressin in patients with portal hypertension: advantages of continuous infusion. J Surg Res 18, 113-117, 1975.

Thorn NA. Present day concepts concerning the release of oxytocin and vasopressin. Ginekol Pol 45, 927-928, 1974.

Thorn NA, Russell JT, Robinson ICAF. Factors affecting intracellular concentration of free calcium ions in neurosecretory nerve endings. In *Calcium Transport in Contraction and Secretion*, pp 261-269, eds F Carafoli, F Clementi, W Drabikowski, A Margreth, North-Holland Publishing Co, 1975.

Thorn NA, Russell JT, Vilhardt H. Hexosamine, calcium and neurophysin in secretory granules and the role of calcium in hormone release. Ann NY Acad Sci 248, 202-217, 1975.

Tissot-Berthet MC, Reinharz AC, Vallotton MB. Radioimmunoassay of neurophysin I and II in human plasma. Ann NY Acad Sci 248, 257-271, 1975.

Tomas T. ADH release from cut pituitary stalk and intact pituitary gland during amygdala stimulation at various frequencies in rats. Neuroendocrinology 17, 139-146, 1975.

Torp-Pedersen C, Thorn NA. Acute effects of lithium on the action and release of antidiuretic hormone in rats. Acta Endocrinol Kbh 73, 665-671, 1973.

Toursal F, Fontaine G. Un analogue synthetique de la vasopressine (DDAVP). Interet dans la traitment des diabete insipides pitressino-sensibles. Nouv Press Med 4, 190, 1975.

Traczyk WZ. Substance P and vasopressin release from incubated in situ posterior pituitary lobe in rats. Bull Acad Pol Sci Ser Sci Biol 22, 731-736, 1974.

Trust PM, Brown JJ, Chinn RH, Lever AF, Morton JJ, Padfield PL, Robertson JJS, Ireland JT, Melville ID, Thomson WST. A case of hypopituitarism with diabetes insipidus and loss of thirst. Role of antidiuretic hormone and angiotensin II in the control of urine flow and osmolality. J Endocrinol Metab 41, 346-353, 1975.

Uhlich E, Haselbeck R, Weber P. Prostaglandin-stimulated vasopressin release from isolated rat neurohypophysis. Acta Endocrinol Kbh Suppl 193, 131, 1975.

Uhlich E, Weber P, Groschei-Stewart U, Roschlau T. Radioimmunoassay of arginine vasopressin in human plasma. Hormone Metab Res 7, 501-507, 1975.

Urry DW, Walter R. Proposed conformation of oxytocin in solution. Proc Natl Acad Sci USA 68, 956-958, 1971.

Vandeputte-Van Messon G, Peeters G. Effects of intraventricular administration of cholinergic drugs on water diuresis in goats. Arch Int Pharmacodyn Ther 211, 80-98, 1974.

Vandesande F. Identification of vasopressin-neurophysin producing neurons of the rat suprachiasmatic nuclei. Cell Tissue Res 156, 377-380, 1975.

Vandesande F, Diereck K, de Mey J. Identification of vasopressin-neurophysin II and oxytocin-neurophysin I producing cells in the brain and hypothalamus. Cell Tissue Res 156, 189-200, 1975.

Vandongen R. Inhibition of renin secretion in the isolated rat kidney by antidiuretic hormone. Clin Sci Mol Med 49, 73-76, 1975.

Vaneckova J, Barthova J, Barth T, Krejci I, Rychlik I. Isolation of antibodies to (8-lysine)-vasopressin by affinity chromatography. Collect Czech Chem Commun 40, 1461-1465, 1975.

Van Gemert M, Miller M, Carey RJ, Moses AM. Polyuria and impaired ADH release following medial pre-optic lesioning in the rat. Am J Physiol 228, 1293-1297, 1975.

Van Wimersma-Greidanus TBJ, Bohus B, Wied D de. The role of vasopressin in memory processes. Prog Brain Res 42, 135-141, 1975.

Van Wimersma-Greidanus TB, Bohus B, de Wied D. The role of vasopressin in memory consolidation. J Endocrinol 64, 30P-31P, 1975.

Van Wimersma-Greidanus TB, Bohus RM, Hollemans HJG, de Yong W. A radioimmunoassay of vasopressin. A note on pituitary vasopressin content in Brattleboro rats. Experientia 30, 1217-1218, 1974.

Van Wimersma-Greidanus TBJ, Dogterom J, Wied D de. Intraventricular administration of anti-vasopressin serum inhibits memory consolidation in rats. Life Sci 16, 637-644, 1975.

Vaughan MK, Reiter JR, McKinney T, Vaughan GM. Inhibition of growth of gonadal dependent structures by arginine vasotocin and purified bovine pineal fractions in immature mice and hamsters. Int J Fertil 19, 103-106, 1974.

Verney EB. The antidiuretic hormone and the factors which determine its release. Proc R Soc Lond Biol B 135, 25-106, 1947.

Vizsolyi E, Perks AM. New neurohypophysial principle in foetal mammals. Nature 223, 1169-1170, 1969.

Vollrath L. New trends in vertebrate secretion. In *Neurosecretion, The Final Neuroendocrine Pathway.* pp 276-284, VI International Symposium, eds F Knowles,

L Vollrath, Springer Verlag, NY, 1974.

Vorherr H, Vorherr UF, McConnell TS, Goldberg NM, Kornfeld M, Jordan SW. Localisation and origin of antidiuretic principle in para-endocrine active malignant tumours. Oncolog 29, 201-218, 1974.

Wade JB, DiScala A, Karnovsky MJ. Membrane structural specialisation of the toad urinary bladder revealed by freeze fracture technique. I The granular cell. J Membr Biol 22, 388-402, 1975.

Wagner H, Maier V, Herrman HJ, Frantz HE. Direct measurement of arginine vasopressin in human serum without extraction procedure. Acta Endocrinol Kbh. 78, suppl 193, 130, 1975.

Walter R. Oxytocin and other peptide hormones as prohormones. In *Psychoneuroendocrinology Workshop*, pp 285-294, Conf Int Soc Psychoneuroendocrinology, ed N Hatotani, Karger, Basel, 1974.

Walter R, Ballardin A, Schwartz IL, Gibbons WA, Wyssbrod HR. Conformational studies on arginine vasopressin and arginine vasotocin by proton magnetic resonance spectroscopy. Proc Natl Acad Sci USA 71, 4528-4532, 1974.

Walter R, Hoffman PL. Tentative identification of a binding site of arginine vasopressin to neurophysin. Fed Proc 32, 567, 1973.

Walter R, Shlank H. Differences in the enzymatic inactivation of arginine vasopressin and oxytocin by rat kidney homogenate. Endocrinology 96, 811-814, 1975.

Walter R, Smith ICP, Deslaurirs R. The conformation of oxytocin in dimethylsulfoxide as revealed by carbon-13 spin-lattice relaxation times. Biochem Biophys Res Commun 58, 216-221, 1974.

Walter R, Yamanaka T, Sakakibara S. A neurohypophyseal hormone analog with selective oxytocin-like activities and resistance to enzymatic inactivation: an approach to the design of peptide drugs. Proc Natl Acad Sci USA 71, 1901-1905, 1974.

Waterson JG. Potentiation of vascular responses to catecholamines by POR-8 (3 ornithine vasopressin). J Dent Res 54, Spec No B, B63-67, 1975.

Watkins WB. Neurosecretory neurons in the hypothalamus and median eminence of the dog and sheep as revealed by immunohistochemical methods. Ann NY Acad Sci 248, 134-152, 1975.

Watkins WB. Presence of neurophysin and vasopressin in the hypothalamic magnocellular nuclei of rats homozygous and heterozygous for diabetes insipidus (Brattleboro strain) as revealed by immunoperoxidase histology. Cell Tissue Res 157, 101-113, 1975.

Walton KG, De Lorenzo RJ, Curran PF, Greengard P. Regulation of protein phosphorylation and sodium transport in toad bladder. J Gen Physiol 65, 153-177, 1975.

Weinstein H, Bern RM, Sachs H. Vasopressin in blood. Effect of hemorrhage. Endocrinol 66, 712-718, 1960.

White MG, Fetner CD. Treatment of the syndrome of inappropriate secretion of antidiuretic hormone with lithium carbonate. N Engl J Med 292, 390-392, 1975.

White RJ, Woodings DF. Impaired water handling in chronic obstructive airways disease. Br Med J 2, 561-563, 1971.

WHO. Expert committee on biological standardisation, 26th report. WHO Tech Rep Ser 565, 18, 1975.

Wirz H. The location of antidiuretic action in the mammalian kidney. In *The Neurohypophysis.*, pp 157-156, ed H Heller, Butterworths, London, 1957.

Wolff J, Alazard R, Camier M, Griffin JH, Cohen P. Interactions of bovine neurophysins with neurohypophyseal hormones. J Biol Chem 250, 5215-5220, 1975.

Yesberg NE, Henderson M, Budtz-Olsen OE. The effect of starvation on water, solute and vasopressin excretion in Merino sheep. IRCS Med Sci 3, 245, 1975.

Yoshida S, Saito T, Murase T. Control of vasopressin secretion. In *Neuroendocrine Control,* pp 189-204, eds K Yagi, S Yoshida, Wiley, NY, 1973.

Young TK, Huang WC. The minimum quantity of vasopressin in the neurohypophysis necessary for water balance in nonstressed rats. Aust J Exp Biol Med Sci 52, 833-840, 1974.

Zimbler H, Robertson GL, Bartter FC, Delea C, Pomeroy T. Ewings sarcoma as a cause of the syndrome of inappropriate secretion of antidiuretic hormone. J Clin Endocrinol Metab 41, 390-391, 1975.

Zimmerman EA, Carmel PW, Husain MK, Ferin M. Tannenbaum M, Frantz AG, Robinson AG. Vasopressin and neurophysin. High concentrations in monkey hypophyseal portal blood. Science 182, 925-927, 1973.

Zimmerman EA, Defendini R, Sokol HW, Robinson AG. The distribution of neurophysin-secreting pathways in the mammalian brain: light microscope studies using the immunoperoxidase technique. Ann NY Acad Sci 248, 92-109, 1975.

Zimmerman EA, Kozlowski GP, Scott DE. Axonal and ependymal pathways for the secretion of biologically active peptides into hypophysial portal blood. In *Brain-endocrine Interaction II.* The Ventricular System. pp 123-134, 2nd Inst. Symp Schizuoka, eds KM Knigge, DE Scott, H Kobayashi, S Ishii, Karger, Basel, 1974.

Zimmerman EA, Robinson AG, Husain MK, Acosta M, Frantz AG, Sawyer WH. Neurohypophysial peptides in the bovine hypothalamus: the relationship of neurophysin I to oxytocin, and neurophysin II to vasopressin in supraoptic and paraventricular regions. Endocrinology 95, 931-936, 1974.

INDEX